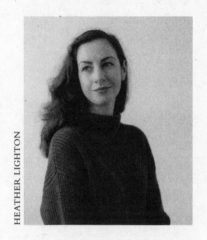

HEATHER LIGHTON

Jessica Friedmann
THINGS THAT HELPED

Jessica Friedmann was born in Melbourne in 1987, and lives in Canberra with her husband and son. She holds a B.A. (Hons) in creative writing from the University of Melbourne, where she received the R. G. Wilson Scholarship, and is a former winner of the Doris Leadbetter Poetry Cup. She has worked as an editor at the independent Australian journals *Going Down Swinging* and *Dumbo Feather*, and her essays, criticism, and feature writing have appeared widely. *Things That Helped* is her first published book.

THINGS THAT HELPED

THINGS

ON
POSTPARTUM
DEPRESSION

THAT

HELPED

Jessica
Friedmann

FSG ORIGINALS ▪ FARRAR, STRAUS AND GIROUX ▪ NEW YORK

To my mother, as promised

FSG Originals
Farrar, Straus and Giroux
175 Varick Street, New York 10014

Copyright © 2017 by Jessica Friedmann
Published by arrangement with Scribe Publications, Australia
All rights reserved
Printed in the United States of America
Originally published in 2017 by Scribe Publications, Australia
Published in the United States by Farrar, Straus and Giroux
First American edition, 2018

Owing to limitations of space, all acknowledgments for permission to reprint
previously published material appear on page 263.

Library of Congress Cataloging-in-Publication Data
Names: Friedmann, Jessica, 1987– author.
Title: Things that helped : on postpartum depression / Jessica Friedmann.
Description: First American edition. | New York : Farrar, Straus and Giroux,
    2018. | Originally published: Things that helped : essays. Melbourne,
    Australia : Scribe Publications. 2017. | Includes bibliographical references.
Identifiers: LCCN 2017038315 | ISBN 9780374274801 (paperback) |
    ISBN 9780374717827 (e-book)
Subjects: LCSH: Postpartum depression—Patients—Australia. | Depression
    in women—Patients—Australia.
Classification: LCC RG852.F75 2018 | DDC 618.7/600994—dc23
LC record available at https://lccn.loc.gov/2017038315

Designed by Richard Oriolo

Our books may be purchased in bulk for promotional, educational, or
business use. Please contact your local bookseller or the Macmillan
Corporate and Premium Sales Department at 1-800-221-7945, extension
5442, or by e-mail at MacmillanSpecialMarkets@macmillan.com.

www.fsgoriginals.com • www.fsgbooks.com
Follow us on Twitter, Facebook, and Instagram at @fsgoriginals

10 9 8 7 6 5 4 3 2 1

CONTENTS

Maribyrnong   3

Pho   7

Red Lips   18

Swanlights, *Turning*   34

Skywhale   67

Center Stage, *Five Dances*,
and Other Dance On-Screen   81

Altered Night   101

Weaving   126

Virginia's Scarf   145

Walking   169

Rings   213

Ainslie   239

NOTES   255
ACKNOWLEDGMENTS   261

THINGS THAT HELPED

MARIBYRNONG

IN THE BEGINNING there was the river, wending its way around the top of the suburb, then snaking out protectively toward the south. The water was deep and cold and full of silt, and in the months after I had my baby I would often dream of going down to drown myself in it.

At dusk the river's parklands were beginning to empty out, the cyclists and joggers wary of the cold and the settling night. Old men who squatted on their heels reeled their fishing lines in, carrying their lures home in scrubbed-out paint buckets. Soon it would be dark; soon a cloistering silence would descend on the leaves and grass, broken only by the rustle of the wind and the steady drone of the highway, as persistent as seawater or the beat of a heart.

I thought of the water as I listened for the baby's breath,

in and out, lightly broken sometimes by a hiccup or a snore. We had made the walk to the river's banks a hundred times over the summer, Mike sometimes breaking off for a run while I saw how many native grasses I could name. Now, in the deep of winter, it ran through my thoughts nightly, bringing a cool little rush with it, a rush of relief. We kept the heating on at home, trying to fend off the drizzle and damp, and ran it through the night "for the baby's sake," though in truth he seemed all right—a hot little furnace running hotter in his sleep.

Through the tide of hormones surging within my body, and the little runnels of blood, and the sour tang of my breasts, I lay awake, listening, and thinking of breath and of water. I had broken my relationship with sleep; it was no longer safe. If I did drift off, the baby's shrills of noise let down my milk and sent a hot flush of sweat through my body before my brain had a chance to catch up, and I would wake sticky and panicked and sure that something was wrong. The sickening wrench of waking was awful, so I lay in bed playing possum; it was better to be passive, to let the baby suckle me without protest and then settle him down to fall asleep again, his small fists raised above his head. I lay awake and listened to the quality of the silence change.

When I was sure the house was asleep again I rolled to the side of the bed gently, so as not to aggravate the incision site, and maneuvered myself up. It was the same move my midwife had taught me, a kind of slow roll-and-rise that made up for the lack of a core. The rest of the house was dead at night, the only center of breath our stale, fecal bedroom, where the heat coalesced and cushioned us into a relentlessly interrupted stupor. Outside the door, which I gently closed, the air was fresh and cool.

The floorboards sent chills upward as I shuffled down the hall. Through the living room, our paintings and books veiled in shadow; past the dining table, smothered in vases of congratulatory flowers. The tiles of the bathroom floor felt like ice against my skin, and I stripped off my T-shirt, soaked with the night's flushes of sweat, and pressed my bare back more firmly against them.

Here, in the quiet, there was only my breath and the rustle of leaves outside. The nauseating heat of my skin, the clamminess of it, found its counterpoint; my breath sounds were the noises of one person, not three. In the cold and calm I lay on my back and thought about the river.

It wasn't hard to draw its coolness around me, its chill. The fog of sleeplessness cohered into a single vision: I would walk out of the house, and cross the highway, leaving no sign behind me. Down the steep hill that led to the river's banks, my hands would reach out for leaves and flowers, touching all the glossy, dew-specked marks of winter growth. Then I would slip out of my clothes, fold them neatly, and disappear beneath the surface of the water.

In a few hours the sun would come up, glinting off the mineral bits of rocks, and discarded fits, and discarded fish-hooks. The oars of boats would shatter the river's surface into a million green-brown sequins, and the new day of its life would begin. The flowers would open to the sun, starved for light. And Mike would wake, and know that I was gone.

He would grieve; I knew he would grieve, but he would be anchored to the earth by this tiny mewling child I felt no stirring of warmth for. He would find love again, because he was easy to love, and another woman would blossom toward our baby and reveal herself to be the real, true mother—the mother our baby would need.

In the cold rush of water my flesh would loosen, become swollen. My engorged breasts would leak a trail of warm milk into the river, the healing wound below my waist be riven in two again, the stitches dissolved. My hair would wash out like weeds, and my eyes would not turn into pearls, but be perpetually turned to the sky.

I knew that it would not be gentle, that it would be violent and raw, but in the midst of the water filling my burning lungs, and the quick blacking out of vision, I would move sideways, catch myself right before death, exist as the slow play of light on the water and the soft rain spattering my growing child when he came to explore the park. In this way I could keep him forever, watching from the reeds.

In the bathroom, collapsed between clusters of night feeds, the vision was compelling. I would wait, and then I would rise again, this time with purpose, and walk out to greet the night, and walk down the quiet hill, leave my body behind, and gently disappear.

I wanted to do it; I was resolved, I had made up my mind. The only problem was that I couldn't get up off the floor.

PHO

BY THE TIME we move to Footscray, Owen is a secret seed, secret even from me. All the time he is there, as I lug cardboard boxes, and scrub paint from sinks, and paint the rental we are leaving a dingy shade of beige—the same shade that, on moving in, we had painted over in pale, pale celery green. It is too early for a rising tide of nausea to clue me to his existence. He is simply, secretly, there.

Almost from the minute that Mike and I begin seeing each other, we talk about our child, the child we will one day have. It should seem much too soon, but nothing feels more natural than lying in the sun at the park, drinking coffee and eating warm bread rolls from the bakery, sketching out our future plans: running a B&B in rural Hungary if I sort out my citizenship; traveling to Berlin; living on a vast property deep in the mountains. And always with a baby in tow.

Our child will be called Coralie, after my great-aunt, or maybe Ivy; Gabriel for a boy. When we get married the fantasies drop away, but the longing for a child remains. We manage to postpone the craving throughout my honors thesis; Mike enrolls in a master's; we do everything we can to pace ourselves, to not jump in, not give in to this deep, visceral craving for the milky smell of a newborn's scalp until, at last, we do give in. It is a surprise to me how much I want a baby, and unbeknownst to me, unpacking boxes in our beautiful new terrace in Footscray, I am hiding the beginnings of one.

Counting backward, I work out that Owen must have been conceived at or just after Rosh Hashanah, the Jewish New Year. New Year, new life: it should be an augury, but I am too nervous to invest the pregnancy with any special symbolism or significance. All I want, when I learn the news, is to make it through to Christmas, six weeks away; for this small ball of matter to become robust and staunch and truly embedded in the lining of his small but swelling home, and then I will believe it; then I will breathe out.

I have always wanted to guard the things I find precious, and in this way I am not good at sharing. I am superstitious: believing in it too much, *wanting* it too much will inevitably mean that I will lose this pregnancy, I think, though to the best of my knowledge I have not lost one before. I have suspected a loss, and that felt aching and raw; and in a small way I grieved it, and it was real grief. I feel like a village woman telling her neighbor their new child is ugly, so as not to draw the attention and jealousy of God.

The morning I suspect I might be pregnant I take a test, and then wipe it clean and carefully bring it into the bedroom, rousing Mike.

"Does this say what I think it says?"

Mike looks at the test and its firm pink declarative line.

"We're having a baby," he says groggily, and pulls me into his arms. Somehow, even knowing this, the day continues as usual. It is not until a work trip to Tasmania the next week, on which Mike has accompanied me and where we camp high up in the mountains, that the fact begins to sink in for him with any clarity and brilliance.

"We're having a *baby*!" he hollers to the ferns in the fern gully, where we have tramped along a rough dirt track. The air is richly oxygenated from the lush green foliage, the forest floor dense with scuttling creatures in the undergrowth; spiderwebs hold drops of moisture, and the night-dark earth seems fertile enough for anything dropped there to take root. Mike grips my hand tightly when we pick our way down the rocks, promising a steady landing.

He wants to tell people when we return, but I hold to my Christmas deadline, superstitious and self-imposed. I have felt the faint tremors of quickening, but I only let my breath out properly much later, at our second ultrasound, when we first glimpse the shape of our child. The ultrasound technician guides the probe around adeptly, angling it lightly into the small hill of my jellied stomach, leaving out identifying details at first, in case we don't wish to know them.

"Do you want to find out the gender?" she asks.

Sex, I silently correct, and then, "Yes."

A slight twist of the probe and then there he is, revealed, tucked up into himself with the small outreaching shadow of his five fingers making a whole hand, a whole hand we can see. The little girl I am half convinced I am carrying floats away and instead, waving from the deep, is this new and unknown thing—a little boy.

As we inch toward Christmas, and the weather gets hotter and drier, each week of viability feeling like a clandestine accomplishment, the nausea becomes more intense. I find out, for the first time, about food aversions, which are much stronger and more visceral than any of my cravings. The provisions I had thought would carry me through my pregnancy—licorice and pickles and dark chocolate and potato chips—are too oily, too salty, too acidic by turns. The only thing I want to eat is pho.

I lie anchored to the couch, moored against the sticky leather with the dry pages of an Agatha Christie novel rustling in the wind, which comes in sudden rushes through our open windows, while Mike traipses up to our local restaurant, Hien Vuong Pasteur. The main drag of Footscray is lined with Vietnamese restaurants, interspersed with relics of the past, like Cavallaro, the pastry shop, or, farther down, Sudanese and Ethiopian food. The competition for best pho is fierce, but we have found our local and are loyal customers.

"For your wife?" the owner asks when Mike comes in, and Mike nods, and soon he is home with two plastic containers, one full of slightly gelatinous rice noodles topped with thin slices of chicken, and the other of rich chicken broth. A little plastic bag of sliced chili, Vietnamese mint, bean shoots, and lemon rounds out the meal, and I carefully pour out half the broth and noodles into a saucepan, and put the rest in the fridge, a safeguard against the next day's nausea.

It is nice to be known. Every morning I walk to work past the Little Saigon market, angling past men in aprons and gum boots unloading their trucks from the fish market, and every morning the sight of glossy-eyed trout and snapper and bream brings a wave of muggy heat up beneath my skin.

I think of my growing child, due in July. He will be a Cancer: a cavorting little crab.

I have never believed in astrology, but now I become avid about the signs, trying to prophesy our future child's personality. Mike is an Aries, I a Capricorn: private, creative, stubborn, the charts say. An earth sign. It is true that I need to walk into the back garden and plant my feet in the cool grass of an evening, watching the sky change color, from parched blue to an industrially shocking pink and then to a pale apricot gray. I am greedy for the sunset. At dusk, the suburb smells like eucalyptus and fish sauce.

We see in the new year at a writer's house in Brunswick, newly built upon a tiny patch that she and her partner have bought, requisitioned from someone's backyard. Though the house is complete the garden is still unfinished, and we stand in a dugout patch among uncovered pipes, as music blares and the sky fills with fireworks. The pregnancy is still hidden, though I think that I can feel my stomach swell, just the smallest bit, beneath the cool and slippery fabric of my dress. Mike puts his hands on my stomach as our friends clamber to the top of our host's old van, shrieking their midnight exhilaration into the sky.

Dead sober and glowing with sweat, I straggle home-ward with Mike at three a.m., losing my favorite lipstick along the way. When we finally find a taxi it first takes us south, then out west. Melbourne is a city split by a river—the Yarra—and people talk of North and South, but now we are heading into a new terrain, demarking a point toward which the compass hadn't already swung in our three years and four houses together. Home.

I had fallen in love with Footscray years earlier, schlep-ping out from Brunswick for a contract stint at Lonely Planet, feeling immediately calmer as I walked down to the banks of the Maribyrnong. My grandparents used to have a shop here, *schmatte*, in the suburb's first wave of migration, before the Europeans ebbed and the Vietnamese flowed, and then the Sudanese, Ethiopian, Congolese, Somali. My grandparents left when a pig's head turned up on their doorstep; the meaning was unmistakable. Nonetheless, I came back, and I loved it.

Sometimes I feel a twinge of guilt; Mike and I and the friends who begin to move westward cannot avoid that *we* are the harbingers of change, the crest of a wave of gentrification that will soon firmly crash, driving house prices upward and longtime residents out of their homes, and closing us all out when rents soar beyond our means. I walk around every room of the terrace ritualistically, blessing our books, our paintings, our spoons, our secondhand furniture, the gold metallic fringe we have hung around our low-hanging light fixtures. We call them "disco chandeliers," and Mike's head brushes through the fringe if he forgets to look where he is walking, but the long strands glimmer as they move in the afternoon light.

Owen ripples and flexes. The curve of my stomach is not hidden now; it pushes insistently outward, the only place I carry any weight until my eighth month, when my face suddenly balloons. I order a few maternity skirts early on, a pair of jeans, trying to get through the pregnancy as cheaply as I can.

When my own birthday passes and the nausea drops away, Mike and I wander down to Hien Vuong to sit together in the window and watch the world pass. Tet, the Vietnamese New Year, fills the streets with neon lights, and wild noise, and smells that wind together on the breeze, so that hints of pho are caught up in the doughiness of *bao* and the oil of Korean Swirl Potato, a newly invented "traditional" snack like a potato cake on a stick. I exult in these smells, which no longer hold the power to upset my balance. It is the Year of the Dragon now: magnanimous, imperious, strong.

I talk to the hospital psychiatrist once a fortnight, trying to gird myself for what might come next. Because I have a history of depression and anxiety, this feels like a sensible step, but I am giddy with joy over the pregnancy, and the shadow side of it doesn't touch me. These fifty-minute hours feel like homework; virtuously completed, but at base unnecessary. At work a colleague laughs when I suddenly swing around, my stomach appearing like an optical illusion from my otherwise unchanged frame.

The weather becomes cooler, the days shorter. Mike turns twenty-nine, and we hold a celebration at our favorite Ethiopian joint, Lucy, named after a famed ancestral hominid also known as Dinknesh. Afterward we all retreat to the house, where a list of names is inked up on thick paper on the wall:

Gabriel
Theodore
Owen
Henry

and one other name I cannot now remember.

"We should vote!" my friend Juliet crows, and suddenly people are passing around bits of chopped-up paper, folding them and dropping them into a plastic mixing bowl. "Teddy" is my choice—a beautiful little boy. Mike is determined, has held the secret knowledge all along, that our child will be named Owen, and when the papers are returned, "Owen" is the winner. I don't know whether the votes have been rigged. It is Mike's birthday, and he gets his wish, and soon I cannot think of our little crab as being anyone else.

The suburb is quieter now in the mornings, the cool air misting over the concrete. A monk stands outside the market, a brass bowl in his hand. In the gray of early hours, he looks like a human marigold, puncturing the gloom with his saffron robe and hi-vis-orange socks.

As the cold creeps in I stew for hours in the bath. Mike comes into the bathroom periodically with a kettle of boiling water to top up the heat, after the gas runs out. Occasionally, he will come in and sit on the floor, playing his guitar and drinking a beer, his jumper sleeve pulled down over his hand when he touches the bottle.

My stomach rises higher and higher over the bathwater, until I can no longer submerge it. My immense breasts float like islands, connected by an atoll beneath the surface. Like Archimedes, I displace more and more water.

Mike is in the kitchen, boiling the kettle.

"Mike. Mike!" I yell.

He runs in, panicked, and then stares in wonder as he sees for the first time our baby's little foot, kicking against my skin, and making the shape of my smooth stomach buckle and distort.

Owen arrives in the bowels of the year, the dreary cold that seems to last forever. He arrives on a Wednesday, which the nursery rhyme prophesies will mean a life filled with woe; as the hospital reminds me, I am predisposed to woe.

He is eighteen months old when we pack up the boxes again; when we take the art off the walls and wrap it in bubble wrap and, when the wrap runs out, clean tea towels and faded pillowcases. We take the fringe down from the lights, and soap off the grimy residue that the double-sided tape has left. It is stiflingly hot again, a new January, Janus-faced. I am a January baby, Janus-faced myself.

We turn ourselves around and orient ourselves toward the east, away from the river and toward the salt of the ocean, St. Kilda, where my parents live, and where Mike and I have lived before. This is where my grandparents, and my father, got off the boat, my grandfather declaring that once he stood on dry, unheaving land he wouldn't go a meter farther. That is the story and it is probably untrue, but I recognize the impulse: to plant yourself firmly in one place and become immovable as stone.

I think of consulting tea leaves, but in truth, they look just like tea. In truth, it is months since I have made up a pot, boiling the water and then letting it cool, rinsing out a cup, sitting in one place long enough to enjoy it. And the magic of augury has waned. I have never believed with more than half a heart in revelations, but I am not sure now whether I am more concerned that they will or will not come true. For the child at my feet, forcing me to sip tea out of a mug over the sink, is not a little crab at all. He is something much stranger and more terrifying and profound, a creature made of my fear and flesh and bone.

RED LIPS

MY SON OFTEN watches me put on makeup in the morning, sitting on the floor while I peer at myself in the mirror. It's a short procedure, but one that keeps him engrossed, because there is a chance I might reach down and swipe him on the nose with my powder brush. Sometimes he grabs a comb as I brush my hair and passes it clumsily through his short locks. "Bruss bruss bruss," he says, satisfied.

In the mirror my face dissolves, swimming back into view as a series of parts: eyes, nose, chin. I dab concealer carefully onto blemishes and pat it dry, sweeping powder over the top in large, loose circles. I pencil in the bit of my eyebrow touched by a scar, balance out my brows for fullness. Then three quick swipes of lipstick—so swift and mechanical that my hand might be autonomous—and my mouth emerges in vivid focus.

In the bathroom cabinet, my lipsticks occupy the highest shelf. Owen is delighted with the transfer of color to material surface; paint onto paper, Texta onto wall. The few times he has found a tube, housing the tomato-orange of Mummy's smile, he has tilted his head, uncapped the tube, and dragged rich, incongruous color across his rosebud mouth in exact mimicry of my gestures. I keep my lipsticks up high because they are expensive, and because of the eeriness of seeing my own expression played out on my small child's face.

The lipsticks that I own are steeped in sex and blood. In my collection, I have Lady Danger; Relentlessly Red; Good to Go. *Cosmo* tells me early on that the painted mouth is supposed to evoke the labia, voluptuous and slightly parted, and the names of my lipsticks bear this out: they are unequivocal. There are fast cars, danger, and passion. There is fire, lust, anger, poppies, roses, all of them packed into small, dark tubes.

I wonder what my child sees when he looks at me in the mirror.

I have worn lipstick since long before he was born; every day, for many years. I can't remember, though, when habit became ritual. I feel as though if I *could*, if I could pin down the moment that commenced a daily ceremony, I might demarcate between girl and woman with clear, metaphoric ease. But when and how do you become a woman? It is a long, raw process that doesn't seem to end.

At thirteen—unlucky number—I become aware that my body is treacherously feminine, by which I mean: *no longer self-contained*. My lithe, sturdy child's frame stretches out inelegantly, and my feet grow sizes and sizes. My skin, previously a trusted vessel for keeping me *in*, erupts into blotches and sores; my thighs and small breasts are lacerated with deep purple stretch marks. In the toilets at school, I begin to bleed.

After that first thin trickle of brown blood, I do not know with any certainty where my body ends and the world begins. In Sex Ed we talk about *penetration*, as though the body is simply a discrete article to be impaled by another, but the soft flesh below is both inside and out, and no one can tell me where in my body I am. Skin turns to membrane, hair to viscous discharge, and I become newly, dangerously permeable.

I have gone through lipsticks and lipsticks, trying to determine which ones will stay on throughout the day; which are too drying; which will erase themselves from the inside out, leaving a raw pink blossom at the center of my mouth. You could chart the last decade by subtle modulations of gloss and color, tiny variations in the pigment of undertones.

When we decide to have a baby I begin to dread my own blood. Ironic—for so long a gush of fresh red was a relief. Now I look at the toilet bowl with deep resentment each month, as though it is holding a loss.

I know that it will take time, that months might pass before implantation is successful. Six months or a year—six or thirteen small chances. I have been on the pill for ten years and don't yet know, coming off, about the cluster of cysts on my left ovary that made me irregular as a teenager. At the time I thought that this irregularity was ordinary, that it was just my body not knowing yet how to regulate itself into neat twenty-eight-day cycles. I had perfect faith in my body working exactly as the Sex Ed pamphlets said that it should.

Now, trying to conceive, it seems that there may be many fewer than thirteen chances in a year; I have downloaded an app on my phone in ignorance, trying to outsmart my body, trying to time things perfectly so as not to feel the twinges that grow into spasms, cramps that begin deep in my womb and wrap around to the lower back so that it feels as though my kidneys are being pummeled.

I hate my body for sloughing off my richest asset, this unwanted endometrium. I eat steak and take iron pills. I want to hoard all of this blood, so rich and precious, and cushion all my hope with it. I stop drinking, in anticipation, and then get plastered each time the toilet water turns red; a bright red lined with white, the inverse of my mouth.

After sex, Mike cradles my belly, astounded at the alchemy that might be taking place. I am still astonished to see myself as beautiful in his eyes, not just for who I am but also for what my body can do. The story of my beauty I am not interested in—I grew up, I shed my adolescent skin, I grew into my nose. My body holds a kernel of possibility that is much richer than anything seen with the naked eye.

I wonder what I will tell Owen when he asks about how babies are made—when, in a few years' time, he hears playground rumors and cutesy, misconstrued facts. I imagine he will squirm with horror, realizing what his father and I have done. But will he feel it deep in his bones, a premonition of what his own body will one day be expected to do? There is a schism looming in our experiences of childhood: he will never feel the fury and revulsion of realizing that his body will have to break open if ever he wants a child. I look at his soft white skin in the bath, his sex organs so casually on display. I kiss his protruding belly as I lift him out. He will always be preciously, casually intact.

• • •

After the blood stops coming my body begins to swell, first adjusting to the feeling of seasickness that holds me pinned to the couch through the stifling December heat wave. At night the temperatures dip below forty, but this provides no relief; in the bathroom, the coolest part of the house, my makeup melts and reconfigures in a tacky approximation of itself. Every morning when I put on my lipstick, I wipe a slick veneer of soupy color from the tip. The color doesn't want to adhere. It mingles with the salt of my sweat, which makes a damp paste of my foundation.

Inside the house I wipe my face clean. My skin surges with hormones, makes me feel like a teenager again. I feel as if any grace or poise I have achieved as an adult has fallen away, and yet I am radiantly happy with my lumbering, swelling self. My breasts are full and large, my belly firmly convex. The tremors I have felt beneath the surface of my skin now resolve themselves into little kicks and hiccups, and then the probing of hands and feet. After seven months I can no longer sleep on my side: the baby pummels the mattress with his tiny fists.

I see my midwife regularly at the hospital, alongside the psychiatrist, and together we make plans that are too firm to ever succeed. I will give birth; I will be healthy; I will love my newborn son.

At thirty-six weeks, Owen flips over in the womb. God knows what prompts him to leave his comfortable, head-down position and somersault upward; it means that my plans change, they have to change. There are only two obstetricians willing to deliver a breech birth vaginally at the public hospital, and there is no guarantee that either of them will be available when my labor begins. Unless the baby resolves the position himself, I will need a caesarean section, officially labeled "elective."

I am ready to push, though; it is so hard to explain. I feel as though the entire pregnancy has been building to this imperative of violence that will retroactively justify the mounting pressures of the body. My midwife recommends yoga, so I stand upside down on my shoulders twice a day, trying to coax the baby into another little spin. Once upside down, I am stuck there, the vast weight of my shifted center of gravity pinning me to the floor. Mike has to help me down, gently, easing me down a bit at a time so that he isn't crushed by a sudden fall. It doesn't help.

I book in for an external cephalic version. On the table I take my skirt off, roll down my maternity tights, and lift my top up to just beneath my breasts. I can feel a little elbow lodged beneath my right ribs, and feet pressing just to the left of my cervix. The baby has been wedged diagonally for a few days now, kicking and hiccuping, defiantly right-way up.

After a few minutes, my midwife beckons in a strong-looking Swedish woman, and a blond student midwife with bright pink gum boots over her scrubs.

"What's with the gum boots?" Mike whispers.

"Delivery room," I hiss back.

The Swedish doctor chats with us as she gives me an injection to relax my uterine muscles. Lying on my back, I can feel but not see the skin of my belly loosening, draping softly over the baby like bread dough over a rolling pin.

An external cephalic version sounds officiously medical, but what it amounts to is this: a strong Swedish doctor will try to turn your baby around from the outside of your body. I grip Mike's hand as waves of pain and nausea ripple up my spine. I stare at the ceiling; Mike watches, wide-eyed, as our little boy is revealed line by furious line, resisting the turning hands with all of his surprising strength.

After the ECV fails, the registrar is supposed to book the C-section, but for some reason doesn't. For two weeks I call my midwife at odd hours, trying to figure out what is happening. She has a habit of repeating back everything I say to her; I don't know if it is a personal habit, a tic, or a professional strategy for making me feel *heard*, but it drives me up the wall. I try not to say anything, as she is so lovely and tiny, but my frustration tolerance is rapidly diminishing as the anxiety begins to spike.

"Katie, I'm really not sure what's going on at the moment—"

"You're not sure what's going on, no—"

"But I really need to *know* when I'm having this baby. What if I go into labor before the caesarean is booked?"

"Go into labor—there's a chance you'll go into

labor—but I'll talk to the registrar again. I don't know why you haven't been booked for an elective section yet."

"I just really need to know. When you find out can you give me a ring?"

"I'll give you a ring."

I sit in the bath every night, displacing monumental amounts of water, and try very hard to remember how to breathe. Mike sits with me, a calming presence in the room. Up until now the pregnancy has been free of panic, though I have been shutting down in the evenings, getting home later and later as work becomes more demanding, and going blank as soon as I am safely through the door.

Panic is a blankness like white noise—those little grains of light in the corner of the eyes, a closing-in of the world. I tell myself it is normal to be anxious; this is a real, not a phantom, source of stress. I am terrified of going into labor and then needing to be cut, of my body getting a taste of what it will not be able to have. I do not want the pain of transition without the catharsis of birth. I do not want this question to remain up in the air, my fate and my baby's dictated by administration and bureaucracy, instead of confidence and foreknowledge and strength.

When the C-section is booked, Mike and I arrive at the hospital with a change of clothes and a few novels packed into a small black leather suitcase, hoping to fit into the day's schedule. I am third or fourth on the list. If there are any complicated deliveries before me, my caesarean will be pushed back to tomorrow or the next day, as I have not, at any point, felt any signs of labor.

Signing into the hospital ward has the same displaced and anticlimactic feeling as waiting in an airport lounge. My sister Claire has a nursing shift at the hospital and comes down for half an hour, keeping us company and joking with Mike. I try not to let the waiting make me tense.

"Can I keep my lipstick on?" I ask the nurse signing me in.

"I don't see why not," she says, laughing at me a little. "You're the first person to ask. Just as long as we can see your fingernails."

I don't laugh. I have stripped off my dress, divested myself of my stockings and underwear and bra. My nude body is covered flimsily by a hospital gown; my hair is tucked up under a baby-blue tissue shower cap. My lips stand out like flames on an otherwise pale face—the last visible sign of any choices I have made on my own behalf.

I have expected hushed lights, maybe soft music, but the room I give birth in is just a room, lined with Laminex cupboards that are filled with drugs. We had planned for walking, stretching, reading, music, and most of all—time. My friend Paulina, living between Poland and Australia, once talked about how much she wished for a long ship voyage, the benefits of a slow transition that are obliterated by flight; she could not believe that you could leave one country, hot and dry and speaking a language full of its own memories and resonances, and wake up a few days later in another land entirely. Here, the fluorescent tubes buzz; I cannot see any natural light.

I walk up a small set of plastic steps to perch on the side of the operating table, then hunch over and part the back of my hospital gown, exposing my spine for the insertion of the spinal block. The motherly woman who has come in to collect the baby's umbilical stem cells—we are donating them—grabs my hands and I wrench them away, furious that anyone but Mike should try to touch me for comfort. He is still standing outside, waiting to be ushered in, entering only when I've been arranged and draped.

The drugs flow up my arm and I start to dip in and out of time.

"Tell me when they've started to cut," I say to Mike.

"They've already started," says the anesthetist with a smile.

Mike sits beside me, holding my unencumbered left hand with his, and stroking my head through the blue tissue cap. Everything sounds a little bit too loud. I struggle to lift my head and see, but it feels too heavy under Mike's soft hand. Then the obstetrician beckons to Mike, and a quick flash of mottled red flesh rises above the curtain separating my breasts from my open belly. It is a monkey of a child, alive in the world at last.

I want to be happy, but the room is beginning to swim. Mike casts a worried glance at me as Katie bustles him out, the bundle of Owen screeching in his arms.

The doctor exchanges a look with the anesthetist, and

then she gets to work. The door to Mike is closed; the pain is ushered in.

I have always paced my breathing, in pain or in times of stress, to the rhythms of T. S. Eliot:

> Let us go then, you and I,
> When the evening is spread out against the sky
> Like a patient etherized upon a table . . .[1]

Usually the words flow around and through me—but when you are that patient? The incantatory magic fails, and I begin to think of Homer, wildly, of the Greeks at Troy slashing long wounds into women so as to rape them through more and more orifices, an unending profusion of cuts. Is it Troy? I am beginning to hallucinate unnatural penetration, the long incision of the scalpel through my belly while my natural causeways, vagina and mouth, are draped and silenced and shut.

And then penetration in reverse—a child coming into the world through unnatural means, blessedly so, so as not to drown in amniotic fluid should the head get stuck, which happens, sometimes, with a vaginal breech—and my baby is alive, not from the bloody gush and tide of passage through the body, but neatly, through this drawing and quartering, a routine procedure, though my fingernails are of their own accord changing color.

I am beginning to hemorrhage.

Fresh blood spills out of me, the color of Russian Red, or Cherries in the Snow. The mantra of a spinal block is "pressure, not pain," but the distinction is semantic. "We're not going to be popular," the obstetrician murmurs under her breath as she and her student begin hurriedly to soak up the bright blood.

Long strips of gauze turn red as the anesthetist tops me up with something that disconnects my mouth from my brain. "Hurt," my brain says, and, "Stop!"

I think of the splashes of bright red, the vivid auras and fragments of Sylvia Plath's tulips. Tulips—two lips. I am beginning to see double.

Underneath my lipstick, my lips are turning blue.

The French word for makeup is *maquillage*, a mask. This isn't so surprising. My grandmother once asked of me, when I came for afternoon tea one day: "Got your face on, have you?" Women of her era *put their faces on*, a daily armor to face the outside world.

This face is the face of femininity, of a performance of womanhood geared toward social acceptance. Second-wave feminists decried cosmetics, which spun out subsequently the term "lipstick feminist," or later, "lipstick lesbian," the lipstick a metonym for all things coded *woman*.

But the mask has a more urgent, more magical property. It is the skin that keeps skin in. Julia Kristeva, the feminist theorist, speaks of the *abject*,[2] that repulsive threat to order, that is neither of the body nor of the world. She gives the example of the skin that forms on the top of a glass of warm milk. She really could just say *skin*: an untrustworthy organ that is both of the body, and not of it, the boundary between the self and everything that threatens it.

Where do I stop, and where does the world begin? Since I first began to bleed, I have not been able to know. When a scalpel slices through the skin at the top of my mons pubis, I do not know. When, later, I grimace as my midwife pulls the metal staples from this gash, which is beginning to knit and heal and close, I do not know.

My uterus becomes so inflamed that it pushes against the scar tissue, a red-hot searing pain. I cannot hold the baby when he is cross, I cannot calm him; if his small foot brushes across the incision site, my vision goes white at this unbearable collision of pressures from both sides. *I have never had a child before*, I reason, I do not know how much pain is "normal." I grit my teeth until the pain makes me behave badly, and the world, for a minute, disappears.

There is a trip to the emergency room.

I lose the next few months in a fog.

There is a fine, powdery shell between me and the world, a shell made of lipstick and pencil and foundation. Where others might see the mask as an indulgence, a dabbling in performative femininity that could be powerfully stripped back for the feminist cause, I cling to it as I cling to everything that holds me together and holds me in.

It is a miracle, to me, that I can defer some of the horror of the abject onto this fragile construction. That my body, this leaking, porous, permeable household of my very shaky subjectivity, can be masked, held, cherished, clothed. Tangible proof that there *is* a barrier to stop me being subsumed is infinitely precious.

Discrete; tangible; self-contained.

Because I'm worth it. Maybe she's born with it. Like flaming diamonds dancing on the moon.

In the bathroom mirror, my face dissolves, and then resolves itself again. My son sits on the floor as I examine the outward signs that I am still all of a piece. Look, there is my nose, hooked and wide, protruding from my face just as it did yesterday, just as it will tomorrow. There is the sweep of my jaw. I send nervous impulses down to my fingertips and concentrate on the texture of my hair as I pile it up, trying to memorize what my body feels like from the outside.

My hands reach out to touch my precious boy, so blessedly coherent when everything else fails. His skin is so soft, so perfect; a few freckles scatter themselves across his nose, and the pink that comes up under his cheeks is rosy and natural and fresh. He grabs my hands as I tickle him, giggles, swats me away.

I open my lips, outline them in pigment. Three quick swipes are all it takes for the consecration of a ritual. All day, in shopwindows, I will catch sight of my vivid mouth, floating in front of my pale, uncertain face, and I will *will* it to open, will my lips to part, to force out some declarative sound, to speak, to give breath and birth to something—to something—but *what*?

SWANLIGHTS, *TURNING*

AT THE TIME that I am writing, we are counting dead women.[1] The year begins when a young Chinese sex worker is murdered in her hotel room, found after the fact with her throat slashed out. It ends when a woman is discovered by welfare officers, battered to death in her home. The feminist collective Destroy the Joint keeps the official score, but all of us, every woman I know, reads of these crimes in the papers and adds a name or a face to her own running tally.

Sometimes the name of a woman is withheld for legal reasons, and we have less than usual to go on to distance her from ourselves. These women are killed at home, at work, in cars, in car parks, in the country, in the city, in the bush; they are killed by strangers, by colleagues, by husbands or ex-husbands or lovers or clients, after being battered or after being raped. When the bodies are found we suck in our breath and think of the keys we hold splayed between our knuckles, makeshift weapons for a lonely walk home.

Sometimes they disappear from the inside of our own small communities. In September 2012, a smiling Irish woman with dark hair and blue eyes appears over and over again on my Facebook feed, where friends and acquaintances anxiously ask if anyone has seen her, and then on the news, when footage is found of the man who may have made her vanish. For six days we wait, hoping defiantly, and then the body is found; abducted from the street where my friend Helen now lives, she has been driven fifty kilometers and buried in a shallow grave. She has been raped and killed, not without putting up a fight, and at the wash of grief emanating from my computer I close the lid and clutch at my newborn child.

I am not the only person I know whose therapist has advised them to turn off the news.

With the outside world at bay I turn and turn, interior. At my core, I keep a resting place for girls and women. Nina Simone resides there, as does Cristina Yang, the painter Helen Frankenthaler, Amy Winehouse, Ruth Park. Closest and most protected and cherished are two artists whose work feels so attuned to the rush and flow of my own thoughts that they feel physically present, sometimes inhabiting my body as ghosts. One is the writer Rumer Godden.

The other is Anohni, once the lead singer of Antony and the Johnsons.

When I first hear Anohni sing, I think for a minute that she might be my older sister. I have always wanted an older sister. I have grown with the idea of a phantom presence hovering a few years ahead of me, someone who could have put her foot on the path first, shown that it was steady and firm, held my hand. It has been in books and music, and history and art that I have found her: someone who reflects me like a mirror set at a slant, familiar but somehow unknown to me, living in my skin.

Listening to Anohni sing, I am astonished to realize that there was a time that I had not yet heard her. It is one of those moments of peripeteia, of vertigo, of something taking flight. I find myself in tears, not just at the beauty of her voice, but at the sense that I have found, as Anne Shirley would say, a "kindred spirit"—not a girlish, plump Diana, but a grown woman whose longing is shot through with loneliness and pain.

Nobody tells you, as a child, that your initiation into womanhood might come at the price of a craving for misuse and violence; that you can protect yourself from others, but that nobody can protect you from yourself.

It is the feeling of being bitten hard on the neck and shoulders; it is the feeling of being held down during sex; it is the longing for obliteration; lust has turned itself inside out and gone feral.

. . .

When I sing to the baby, I make up lines about whatever it is that we are doing at the time. I find the ability to turn on a stream of nonsense striking in its ease; all the little rhymes and lyrics and poems that became part of my own tissue as a child crawl below the surface of my skin like little worms. Snippets of song make their way toward all uses. When I bathe the baby in the laundry sink, I sing

> *Baby in the washing machine*
> *Oh no! He's very clean*

to the tune of "Girlfriend in a Coma," and laugh as he grins at the sound of my voice. His whole body fits diagonally in the deep sink, and he floats happily with my hand behind his neck, keeping his tiny nose and mouth above the water.

Taking the baby for a walk, I meet a young father in the park, whose child is playing on the seesaw. The little boy has only a few years' experience of speech; he sings:

> *Seesaw, Margery Daw,*
> *Johnny shall have a new master.*
> *He shall earn but a penny a day*
> *because he can't work any faster.*

"Where do these songs *come* from?" the man asks, catching my eye with a laugh.

"I think this one is from the Industrial Revolution," I say, "but a lot of them seem to be about the Plague."

"Oh . . . which ones?" he asks, and my mind goes blank. The resurrection of long-buried lyrics only goes in one direction; they can make their own way toward the conscious parts of my mind, but I cannot dig down and retrieve them.

I leave the man and his son behind me as I walk the baby around the curve of the river. When I get home I look for my copy of *The Uses of Enchantment*,[2] but the words fly off the page; already I am losing the ability to read. Online, where things come manageably in dribs and drabs, I find that the rhyme first appeared in print in 1700, and may have been a work song for sawyers, keeping a rhythm steady as their shared saw bit into the wood. There is no such woman as Margery Daw, but in Scots a "daw" is a slattern, and they have another song about her:

> *Seesaw, Margery Daw,*
> *sold her bed and lay on the straw;*
> *sold her bed and lay upon hay*
> *and pisky came and carried her away.*
> *For wasn't she a dirty slut*
> *to sell her bed and lie in the dirt?*

I daydream about sleeping in the garden, on a bed of moss, comfortable and autonomous until a maleficent being carries me away. When I read the news, I don't know what is real and what is fantasy anymore.

• • •

The nursery rhyme that I am trying to think of is "Ring a Ring o' Roses," which is apocryphally about the Black Death. Historians reject this idea, but other rhymes have their feet more firmly in myths and folklores based on historical practices.

"London Bridge Is Falling Down" is supposed to refer to rumors of infants immured in the bridge as a sacrifice to the gods. There is no evidence of bones there, but immurement happened; foundation sacrifices have always been an idiosyncratically accepted practice, as *hitobashira* in Japan, and in Serbia, Hungary, and Romania, where again and again myths make reference to the wife of a wealthy landowner being the one sacrificed to propitiate any evil spirits. It is not just that women are *buried in the earth*; we are also buried in the structures that populate the earth, holding them up invisibly; invisible pillars.

"Margery Daw" goes back to the seventeenth century, probably earlier. In the sixteenth and seventeenth centuries, men still sing sawyering songs; the mechanization of the sawyer's arm is yet over the horizon, caught up in a chain of events that will bring their profession to obsolescence, at least in the West. For thousands of years—since Pliny, Seneca, and Plato laid down their prohibitions against mining—bronze and iron have been the only interruptions to a scheme of agriculture, of permaculture, and of a life that is confined to the surface of the land.

Pliny believes that the earth is endowed with a female

soul, and that to plunge a shaft beneath her skin is akin to rape, a violation that will cause only lust, greed, and avarice in the hearts of men. Men take seriously the idea of "sinning against the earth," though if flashes of gold or fool's gold turn up in a local stream, they will take their pans and roll up their trouser legs and pan for the longing of their hearts. Pliny warns that intercession into the earth will result in earthquakes; they are the natural consequence of the earth's deep displeasure.[3]

Many are fearful, too, to disturb the ecosystem below the earth's surface, which they, like the Ancient Greeks, believe to consist of rich soil in which metal trees grow; the veins of silver and gold that sometimes spit a nugget into the rivers are the tree's branches and leaves. Their roots are in the core of the earth itself, which has formed them from mist; they are as alive as animals and fruit, though of a significantly lower order.

But men cannot leave anything to be still, they cannot seem to leave a thing untouched. It is Agricola, in 1556 in *De re metallica*, who argues for the utility of mining. A fish, he says, is similarly hidden from view, but with human industry and the iron fishhook, can be retrieved from the river and enjoyed as part of nature's bounty. Pliny is overturned, and the popular view of nature goes from being that of a powerful, prevalent mother, imbued with wisdom and mystery, to being merely pasture and field: calm, bountiful, orderly.

I watch a child sing on a seesaw, then head home to research his chants on a device that is connected to vast warehouses of power by cables slung deep beneath the ocean. The scales have been tipped for years, the moment already decided. The earth has been divested of her formerly secret caches of ores, of minerals, sheared of her forests; cycles have been disrupted, fluids made corrupt. We have entered the age of the Anthropocene, where isotopes left by nuclear testing can be found in the rock formations of the Antarctic. Nothing will be untouched by human hands from now on; not a rock, not a leaf, not a skeleton dug deep into the dirt.

Where are women in all this? They are stoking the fires, bearing the children, practicing sorcery in the dark light of the moon. As Agricola and others argue for the innate passivity of the earth, at the edge of Arcadia a shadow-self springs up. If the earth's virtues are femininely passive, to be rewarded, praised, and plundered, so, too, are her storms, her earthquakes, her thundering torrents feminine; they are the darkly transgressive, uniquely female ebbs and flows of a treacherously membranous body. Where the calm, pacific mother lives, there will always be the temptress, the heretic, the witch.

Now it is not just that nature is disordered when it deviates from its subservience to the industry of man—women, heretical women, derive power from its disorder; they control it. They can summon hail from the blue sky, brew plague, send disease skimming across an otherwise healthy crop. Those claiming these powers are sometimes "ordinary" women, as well as anyone who visibly or socially transgresses: the infidel, the disabled, the intersex or transgender woman.

These women do not need the hierarchies of spirituality that the Church clamps down on its faithful. The world is animate; it is imbued with a soul, and trees and squirrels and streams can speak to women, much as its minerals and ores have been calling to men. Some of these women will take up witchcraft actively; others, perhaps a vast majority, are simply troublesome. Whether too carnal, too elderly, with too sharp a tongue, there now exists a helpful and legally sanctioned social category that will strip her of her autonomy, and put her to her death.

Resistance, resistance to hierarchies, stops being necessarily an active endeavor, and instead becomes rooted in the dissonance of bodies, the dissonance of minds. If a woman does not want to pray; if she is not a natal woman, but born with genitalia that deviates from the norm; if she does not celebrate the birth of her child, but mourns instead and turns her face to the wall, then she is likely to be condemned a witch, to die. And if she is already condemned, why not take up the powers and pleasures of control?

Women's bodies have always been a battleground. Carolyn Merchant, in her spectacular book *The Death of Nature*, recounts the physician Johann Weyer's defense of witches, in 1563, which aims to save the lives of women by nonetheless stripping them of physical and intellectual agency:

Women confess to crimes really done by the
devil [he writes] "while their minds are
wounded, troubled, and disturbed by phantoms
and apparitions in brains already addled by
melancholy or by its vapors."[4]

That "melancholy" that Weyer refers to is, of course,
depression. It is the same melancholia that Hippocrates
diagnoses as an illness that encompasses instability in the
humors, particularly the humor of black bile. It is associated with the earth as an element—I keep in mind that
I am a Capricorn—and with coldness, dryness. Long before
the witch trials begin, it is associated with demonic posses-
sion; if melancholia cannot be cured by diet and medicine,
it seems likely that there is something supernatural lurking
just under the skin, rebuffing the best attempts of men to
tame it.

Hippocrates's beliefs about melancholia are concurrent
with the medical understanding that hysteria—a woman's
neuroticism and anxiety, dissociation, psychosis—is caused
by the wandering womb: too light, too dry, a shriveled
womb that has unanchored itself from the vaginal muscle
and is now causing havoc in the body. Here it is putting
pressure on the heart; here it is seeping squelchily through
the intestines.

I try to put myself back in time, to the witch time, and
I find myself incinerated, burning. Symptoms of melancholy and hysteria taken together would almost certainly
have indicated witchhood, or if your priest was generous

about your postpartum inabilities, being under the influence or curse of a witch. For what good, sane, God-fearing woman would rather embrace a stake and bonfire than feed and care for her new, tiny child?

As illness clamps down on my shoulders, music becomes almost intolerable. Any noise feels viscerally assaultive, with the exception of certain string arrangements, one film soundtrack, and Anohni's voice. It is like a harp, it is like whale song, and I need a small core of stillness within me to be able to receive it. With illness pressing down fast, I spend more and more time in the bath, where the hot water is almost scalding and depresses my sympathetic nervous system, and the mist of steam frazzles and curls my hair.

With my baby and husband in another room, with the thin evening light slanting through the window, I feel as though I can inhabit every atom, as if through the pressure of the water and the weight of the song I can hold my body together at least temporarily, not dissolve or fly into pieces. When the anxiety hits I find myself floating outside my own skin, wanting desperately to find a way back inside—but I have never floated above myself in the bath, only resisted the temptation to sink down completely.

Outside the window it begins to drizzle, shutting me in. Anohni's voice coils around the vibration of strings, protecting the sound like the sheath of a nerve:

Her eyes are underneath the ground
I have heard the crying sound
No one can stop you now . . .[5]

But the crying sound is coming from outside the door, and Mike enters the room with a wailing infant, and I rise out of the steam and hold him gingerly to my suddenly leaking breasts, hating them both for interrupting this reverie, this small pocket of time in my day that is psychically and physically bounded only by myself. I am *touched out*; this is what they call it when you have been stroked and suckled and grabbed so much that you cannot bear a second more of physical contact, like a cat that turns vicious out of the blue.

Feeding my baby, I take care not to let his heels dip into the scalding water. Someday, I think, my body *will* fly apart.

Watching ballet videos in bed, an algorithm takes me from Natalia Osipova and Carlos Acosta rehearsing for *Giselle* to a fan video for Anohni's "River of Sorrow." As usual, the words carry me along on a swell of pity:

There is a black river.
It passes by my window
and late at night
all dolled up like Christ

I walk the water
between the piers . . .[6]

The song was written for Marsha P. Johnson, after whom the Johnsons are also named; a tribute to a queer black woman, a fierce activist who threw one of the first bricks at the Stonewall riots and spent her days walking the streets decked in flowers, a mother to lost children, a "saint." I think of Johnson leaving her Santería-influenced offerings to the spirits of the water in the river where her body would wash up in 1992. The police ruled Johnson's death a suicide, and it took twenty years of activist intervention to see the case reopen as a potential murder. But the evidence, by now, has washed away.

There are women in rivers, and women in the earth—*wilis* who have died for love and are rising up and calling out for us. I think, almost constantly now, of the Maribyrnong, its soft, cold silt and the sprouting grass covering the ground like pubic hair at its lip. In some rational corner of my mind I know that suicide is an affront, not just to myself—my self, which is already in danger of splitting up and flying away—but to the thousands of women who end up in rivers not by choice but by violence, who would raise their hands out of the water for a chance to pull me in and take my place.

On good days I try to jeer myself out of it. *Isn't it just like a white woman,* I tell myself, *to think that she can choose to go where so many black, gay, poor, elderly, sick, disabled women have gone unwillingly.* But this jeering isn't laughter—it's a long nail of self-abnegation that I take pleasure in impaling myself on. If I cannot die, then at least I can be pierced with small holes for the wind to whistle through.

The women in the news are nearly always dead. If they are not dead, they have been raped; if they have not been raped, they have been mutilated, and they are speaking up as survivors, survivors of cancer, survivors of violence, survivors of female genital mutilation. We, as women, like women to survive.

Mostly, though, they are dead—either dug up from the ground or killed as fertilizer, in service of it. Honduran environmentalist Berta Cáceres wins the Goldman Environmental Prize and is assassinated, killed in her own home, shot dead by two men for her brilliance agitating for Lenca land rights and for her ferocity in exposing the ecological devastation that has been allowed by the corruption of her government.

She is something like the hundredth environmentalist to be murdered in Honduras in the last four years. Of course she had received warning, she had many warnings, but these days, who doesn't receive death threats? Women I follow on Twitter receive them for speaking out about politics, for telling the stories of their rape, for writing video game reviews. We speak of them in the way we speak of our periods: *When did you get your first?*

For those women who do not menstruate, the threats are exponentially intensified, as they are for women whose bodies flout accepted norms in color, in health, in ability, in scope. We speak of *intersectionality* as though we are describing the two pieces of wood that meet to form the cross upon which we will be hung.

Is it any wonder that when the hierarchy we live with is unknowably cruel, and a place in the "natural" order is denied, strange and transgressive powers spring up? It is not only menses, breast milk, wandering uteruses that cause us to turn to sorcery. Anohni, like Marsha P., is not a natal woman, but a newly born woman, born of difference, and this gives her automatic initiation:

> I'm a witch. I actually de-baptized myself. And
> what's great about being transgender is you're
> born with a natural religion. It applies almost
> across the board; no matter what culture or
> economic group or nation that you're from,
> you're almost automatically a witch. None of the
> patriarchal monotheisms will have you. It's very
> clear that in most of those religions you'd be put
> to death. In many parts of the world you still are
> put to death.[7]

In the parts of the world where one is *not* put to death, the transgender person is often revered as a shaman, with access to both men's and women's knowledge, or the knowledge of the natural world and of animals. The shaman's role is to enter a trance state, commune with spirits, to heal, to sing, to guide newly departed souls into the land of the dead, to divine the future. This is a tradition that dates back to the Stone Age, far preempting Iron and Bronze, and the Neolithic Period.

To inhabit, to channel, to commune; these are the gifts of shamanism and witchcraft, they are the gifts of *flow*. I think of the flow of blood, a monthly tide, or the blood that wells up to sustain the heart and lungs in song. I think of the hypnotic ebb and flow of Anohni's strings and voice, suggestive, transformative, and her heart that encompasses both masculine and feminine aspects of the world; the queerness of it, both queer in the original sense of eerie, and in its joyously contemporary use.

I don't know if I believe in magic. It seems to rely so heavily on perspective. But there is something profoundly powerful in the word made flesh, through music, or song, or a whispered mantra, a secret spell.

Reading Mircea Eliade, I come across the ties between the figure of Mother Earth and the Goddess of Death, birth in another guise: "Death is likened to the seed which is sown in the bosom of the Earth-Mother to give birth to a new plant."[8] All shamans, whatever the culture, are required to undergo an experience that brings them close to death before they are able to acquire their powers; it is an initiation rite.

For many shamans and witches, this journey to the brink of death is a metaphorical journey, a taking leave of the senses—the ordinary senses that keep us tied to the

loamy smell of dirt and the crisp, cool morning breeze—
to travel astrally or psychically along another plane. Those
who return are lauded as having made spiritual sense out
of a period of madness. Those who do not return are simply lost.

Curled up in bed, I watch *Turning*, the documentary that
Charles Atlas and Anohni made after their performance at
the Whitney Biennial in 2004. Two years later, they take
this performance on tour: a circle of thirteen women stand
on a platform, which slowly rotates, as Atlas projects their
faces against the wall, and Anohni performs the early parts
of her repertoire. The film is not released until ten years
after the tour; in the time between then and now, so many
things change, so many stay the same.

These models who are turning are natal and trans
women from all walks of life; they are young, they are elderly, they are unadorned, and sometimes they are overwhelmingly made-up, the artifice overtaking the woman
so that you may at first not know she *is* a woman. In snippets of interview, conducted by Anohni, they talk about
their lives before and after the turning, mostly well before—
when they believed that they lived too untidily outside nor-
mative behavior, that they would either die at somebody
else's hand or give in to the compulsive urge to suicide.

It is astonishing, this project of women bearing witness to one another. One by one, they leave their place in
line, and walk up to the stage, wordlessly supported by a

circle of women who will *see* them, *acknowledge* them, heal invisible griefs. The word that is used is always *sisterhood*—the project deliberately evokes and sometimes replicates the structures of '70s-style feminist consciousness-raising, and Anohni will later convene a symposium, Future Feminism, to raise consciousness of the ecofeminism that permeates her work.

For *Turning*, she flits through here and there, conducting interviews with the performers, and taking Julia Yasuda up the Eiffel Tower in a fuzzy pink jumper; it is the only point in the film at which I cry. Anohni's seemingly innate shyness recedes when she is onstage, in any creative capacity, giving cryptic performance notes to the orchestra and the models; at first these notes are about remembering a time that they felt loved; then:

> Maybe perhaps tonight you could imagine if you're tired, you could imagine that you're actually already dead, and that you're just a skeleton. Let the wind be alive, the wind blowing through your bones. So everything that's dancing through you is elements. It's wind, it's water, it's ice, and snow, and fire. Just elements are blowing through your dead body, your skeleton. So you're just gone completely, you can be asleep.[9]

It is easy to tell from a second of reaction shots who, like me, finds this fantasy incredibly comforting, and who is disturbed. Anohni catches the reactions, too, and calls herself back to a framing of the question as one of imagination:

> So have a lovely—just have a creative adventure,
> you know? Inside yourself.

There is an exquisite sense of relief in imagining oneself as merely a skeleton hung with flesh, exhausted, entranced, and able to survive penetration by water, fire, ice. *Survive* is probably the wrong word for a fantasy about bones; the holes with which I have pierced myself are imaginary, my flesh blocks these elements at all but a sub-atomic level; tiny electrons and protons, rippling through my flesh, as wind, as light, as sound. I close my eyelids and stare at the sun through the window, taking in the nectarine quality of light, the tiny threads of red-blood veins.

For Catherine Clément and Hélène Cixous, French feminists of the sisterhood-circle age, the sorceress has a direct descendant in the hysteric—they are both part of a small group of "women who die for women," as Jesus died for men. In "The Guilty One," Clément writes that this feminine role, the sorceress-hysteric, is liminal and ambiguous, existing outside of hierarchies, but inadvertently serving to enforce them:

> The sorceress heals, against the Church's canon;
> she performs abortions, favors nonconjugal love,

converts the unlivable space of a stifling
Christianity. The hysteric unties familiar bonds,
introduces disorder into the well-regulated
unfolding of everyday life, gives rise to magic in
ostensible reason. These roles are *conservative*
because every sorceress ends up being destroyed,
and nothing is registered of her but mythical
traces. Every hysteric ends up inuring others to
her symptoms, and the family closes around her
again, whether she is curable or incurable.[10]

That last, written in 1975, I find blessedly—and
cruelly—untrue. I am not inuring Mike against my symptoms; he becomes sick with worry, body thickened and
made stiff with the burden of caring for a wife as well as
a child. But I am deeply, sickly aware of "introduc[ing]
disorder into the well-regulated unfolding of everyday life."
If I am accosted with melancholy, possessing the charac-
teristics of a sorceress or the desperate somatic disturbances
of a hysteric, I am a uniquely powerless one, devoid of chant,
trance, control.

Clément goes on:

In *Tristes Tropiques*, Lévi-Strauss distinguishes
two forms of repression (or two forms of
integration, one could say). The anthropoemic
mode, ours, consists in vomiting the abnormal
ones into protected spaces—hospitals, asylums,
prisons. The other, the anthropophagic

mode, examples of which are found especially in ahistorical societies, consists in finding a place for anomaly, delinquency, and deviancy—a place in the sun at the heart of cultural activity. The history of the sorceress oscillates between the two poles and often ends in confinement or in death.

To come out, then, as ahistorical, as deeply ill, as "hysterical," as "melancholy," as shamanic, entails phenomenal risk. There is nothing innate to our status as women on the margins of an "organized" society that guarantees us any particular reception; compassion, disgust, aid, contempt, reverence, revulsion, all spin like a roulette wheel in front of our dizzying eyes. The popular narrative seems to be that shame keeps us quiet about our illnesses, our vulnerabilities, but where there might be shame there is also a very real and pressing threat of danger.

Clement wonders what happened to Emmy von N., as she wonders what happened to Dora, and the many analysands who dropped out of Freud's literature as his interest in hysteria ebbed away; she has already answered her own question. Judith Herman, in *Trauma and Recovery*, tells it more bluntly: after listening brilliantly and empathetically as patient after hysterical patient revealed a past trauma, usually a childhood sexual trauma, Freud repudiated his findings lest the moral code of his entire existence, one that was staked on a sure, responsible patriarchy, be shaken into dust:

His correspondence makes clear that he was increasingly troubled by the radical social implications of his hypothesis. Hysteria was so common among women that if his patients' stories were true, and if his theory were correct, he would be forced to conclude that what he called "perverted acts against children" were endemic, not only among the proletariat of Paris, where he had first studied hysteria, but also among the respectable bourgeois families of Vienna, where he had established his practice. The idea was simply unacceptable. It was beyond credibility.

Faced with this dilemma, Freud stopped listening to his female patients.[11]

Where the sorceress can heal, the hysteric has for centuries leaned against men and found them no prop at all. It is striking that Clément mentions the role of sorceresses in providing abortions; this aspect of witchcraft usually goes well under the radar, but witches, midwives, and "old wives" have run an underground movement in providing women's health care for millennia. Our wombs and our hearts and our minds have been mysteries to men, veiled from their eyes by their own determined obtuseness.

It has only really been for the past twenty years or so that psychiatrists like Judith Herman and Diya Kallivayalil and Bessel van der Kolk have been listening to women, taking the root causes of their trauma seriously, and in doing so realigning hysteria, most commonly now classified in somatic and dissociative disorders, as a reasonable expression of post-traumatic stress.

"Hysteria," as a category, held on as a proper psychiatric discourse until it was removed from the third edition of the *Diagnostic and Statistical Manual of Mental Disorders* (*DSM-III*) in 1980. The establishment is slow to move; complex post-traumatic stress disorder is still very likely to be wrongly classified as borderline personality disorder, moving the root of psychic destruction and the attendant responsibilities for this devastation away from society, and into the bodies of the women themselves.

Postpartum depression is its own thing, of course, not a result of trauma in the clinical sense; straightforward, simple, approachable, it needs no sorceress magic in its treatment and identification. Still, a postpartum onset specifier for major depressive disorder was only added to the *DSM-IV* in 1994, and when I walk into the emergency room in 2012, the people there who are willing and able to help me are almost exclusively women.

When I step out of the bath, the mirror is steamed up, and all I can see is the outline of my body. In this view I am beheaded, for which I am glad. My skin has erupted from all the hormones, the sleeplessness, the cold, and my face is pitted with swelling pustules and the purple scythes of freshly healing scars. When I catch Mike looking at me with concern and love, I turn my face away, humiliated that he should bear witness to my ugliness.

As the mist clears, I can see beyond the outline of my body. I have dropped weight in the past few months, shedding the baby weight until I am back to the contours of my old self, then going beyond this point as I lose interest in food altogether. The baby is voracious, and I have stopped stockpiling little caches of fruit and nuts all over the house; what is the point? Breastfeeding exhausts me, but it is an exhaustion of compliance.

My breasts themselves are swollen, less so after the baby's fed, but still much larger and firmer than anything I am used to. If I squint, if I discount my head, I am shocked by how womanly I look, "womanly" in the sense of full, curved, voluptuous. It is the body I used to daydream about as a teenager, when I was still waiting to develop; it is a perfect hourglass, and it brings me absolutely no sensual pleasure at all. I can look at it, but I feel divorced from it. It is not me; it is only a thing that I am wearing. All I see is how completely my gender resides in my body, and how alien I have become from any of the hedonic powers it is supposed to possess.

What draws me to Anohni, what makes me feel a kinship with her? Without a doubt, it is not just the beauty, it is the masochism. There is a strand of her lyricism that simply and straightforwardly expresses a longing for pain; her female body is mapped onto a suffering earth, and she suffers with it, willingly, complicitly. I am eighteen with a kind, loving boyfriend, slipping in and out of depression, trying to keep to the surface of the water: friendship, love, sex. But I feel like a knife has been turned in my gut the first time I listen to "Fistful of Love":

> I accept and I collect upon my body
> the memories of your devotion
>
> I feel your fists
> and I know it's out of love
> and I feel the whip
> and I know it's out of love
> I feel your burning eyes burning holes
> straight through my heart
>
> It's out of love . . .[12]

or to "Cripple and the Starfish":

> I am very happy
> so please hit me
> I am very, very happy
> so come on hurt me
>
> I'll grow back like a starfish
> I'll grow back like a starfish . . .[13]

I have no explanation for how closely the desire to be hurt hews to my bone. It is not a metaphor, it is a secret fact, one that I have harbored like a strand of rot in my own sensuality since I first started thinking about death.

Sometimes I think it is connected, very simply, to the lifelong flashes of vertigo I have experienced, during which I lace my fingers through the hard diamonds of hurricane fencing at the station so as not to hurl myself in front of a train. How safe, how comforting it would be to have someone, a lover, hold my wrists firmly, close enough to leave a bruise, to keep me from hurling myself toward a void. It is a transfer of responsibility, an abdication: I cherish the scene in *Secretary* where Edward takes away Lee's little pencil case full of razors, and informs her that she will never hurt herself again. It is the most erotic moment in the film, this shift in power.

Perhaps it is a consequence of the threat of violence that we live with daily that we are constantly aware of it, absorb it, learn to love it as people do love their oppressors. We hear men refer to our vulvas as "gashes," as "axe wounds"; no wonder we cannot distinguish violence from sex. And from sex comes forth another splitting of the body—birth, with its intense, transcendent pain and shattering of autonomy. We take classes to remember, simply, how to breathe.

As I listen to Anohni, I wonder if masochism is a viable political strategy, and whether creative collaboration with a force of violence, of oppression, can ever be justified; *at least*, I think, *at least* it gives voice to the victim; it turns an assault into a pas de deux, defusing the violence of the aggressor's intentions in the same way that we reclaim words like *cunt* and *whore* and use them with each other in loving affection. The danger, though, is that you have to internalize them either way. There is a fine, fine line, a cobweb separating this reclamatory masochism from the real, suicidal longing for self-obliteration.

As I walk along the river, I try to blink out the used fits and plastic bags it coughs up. I think about the damage that has been wrought to this part of the earth in just a few hundred years, and try not to think about colony collapse and the death of bees, or the trillions of tiny plastic particles flowing out to the ocean from exfoliators containing "microbeads"; the coal mine that is on fire a hundred kilometers away, and the old-growth forests that are being logged for wood chips in the south.

I cannot find the logic in it; the ongoing devastation of the environment at such a rapid pace defies sense. Each fresh piece of knowledge of the ways in which the earth is being harmed sends me spiraling. When I think of the harm that *I* am doing, simply by existing in a system that seems irrevocably corrupt, I cannot find an ethic for continuing to exist.

I read the pleas of sixteenth- and seventeenth-century scholars against intrusion into the earth, and feel as though I am living in a double time, in all time. I can see the despair and reproach of those scholars, who beg to let the earth be, to put the cycle of nature before the imperative of commerce, and do so with a good working knowledge of what will come if their pleas are ignored; I have seen that same look on the faces of people at climate marches, who vote for Green parties, and write letter after letter on behalf of asylum seekers and refugees: a staunchness in the face of almost certain futility.

The fact that sometimes Anohni's voice flows through me in precise articulation of my griefs and fears, her fierce ecofeminism dignifying the earth, resurrecting slaughtered women, demanding empathy and hope—in these moments, it doesn't move me. It gives the same false assurance that comes from the hospital nurses when they say, "You're not alone, you know. Other women have gone through this." God, as though it's not bad enough that *I* have to! This is how I feel: as though the pain of living is not lessened when shared, but exponentially increased. The grief of other women, of grasses and oceans, is clawing out my belly, begging to be heard.

As I begin to lose touch, violence feels ever closer. Knives glimmer in the sunlight of the kitchen, and I cannot stop the thought of dragging each and every one of them across the inside of my thighs. It is an ugly thought; I think about how the serrated edge of the bread knife must at first make little pinpricks, like the bloody footprints of an ant. Everything feels dangerous—the soft, smothering couch cushions, the glass of water I keep next to the bed, the cord of Mike's dressing gown.

I croon to the baby,

I would die for you, I would be your slave.
My womb's an ocean full of grief and rage . . .[14]

and I wonder how, just *how* this woman, childless and un-known to me except for through her music, has so perfectly described the desperation of my maternity, the bubbling-up rush of the tide.

There is something about the baby's helplessness that brings out a corresponding brutality. I understand for the first time what it is to want to torture something weaker than yourself; to want to hurt. When his crying reaches a crescendo, my anger does, too, brilliant, sparkling, and with it a treacherous sense of vindication: I was wrong to have this child, my disgust toward him is morally just. His vulnerability is all that I can think about.

When I lift him carefully from his bassinet, I take care to support his little neck, but flashing across my mind again and again is an image of the hard square corner of the dresser. His head, still so tender, is fragile, the fontanel like the bruises beneath the skin of a ripe peach. In my mind I seize his neck and bring his head down with one clean gesture, the corner of the table denting deeply into his skull.

When I think of damaging the vulnerable soft spots of his head, the thought is not wished for, but I pay for it as though it has been. And I give thanks that I can; I believe for a minute that this is the *why*. That the walks home alone from the station at night, and the close encounters with drunk and determined men, and the nursery rhymes about women in walls, and the news reports of corpses found in apartment buildings have taught me how to swallow violence, how to digest it. In this moment of danger every unwanted brutal and sadistic thought is seamlessly turned inward, almost with a sense of pleasure, the pleasure of flagellation. It is not by any means the only fantasy I indulge in.

In therapy I will learn that intrusive thoughts are an incredibly common symptom of postpartum mood disorders. When I am well enough to distinguish illness from health, I will resent these flashes of brutality and spite the most; as though it is not enough that I am hollowed out, made dull and gray and self-loathing, without having to pay for it in this deepest of other ways. I will come to see that illness is curdling my ability to love, except through the sacrificial act of subsuming violence, and at the cost of incredible damage to the self.

We joke and laugh and demystify the grotty parts of motherhood—smeared banana on our best pants and credit cards stuck in our computer drives—but we do not talk about these moments: when we dream of running our children under boiling taps or pinching their small noses closed; when the pitch of their constant crying leads us to vivid images of harm; when our rage bubbles over and the thoughts running through our minds are compulsive and unrelentingly terrifying. I wonder how many women *do* realize that these thoughts are a symptom, though so insidious that they feel like *us*, our secret selves. I wonder how many women, shocked at this revelation of their secret capacity for harm, will keep their guilt and shame to themselves, and never allow themselves the opportunity to heal.

. . .

When the baby is three months old, I make a phenomenal effort to leave the house. I dress not in the faded black maternity skirt I have been wearing for months, but in a vintage two-piece set, the top scooped low and edged with a knitted black lace, the waist nipped in with a proper, nonelastic closure. I give myself five minutes more than I need to walk to the train station, and wait with my thumb hooked through the slats of a seat until the train arrives.

In three years Anohni will be in Australia again, but I do not know that now. She will return to perform at MONA, and I will be well by then, blossoming, happy on and off, with a beautiful child and an antidepressant that works, but unable to go to gigs for lack of cash. It is money I would willingly give if I had it; she will give the proceeds of her concert to the Martu people of Parnngurr in Western Australia, to aid in their legal battle against the construction of a uranium mine on country.[15] There seems no end to things fought over and dug out of the earth.

Later still, she will shed her natal name of Antony and appear as Anohni, fiercely political, putting her dirges to the side. "I have grown tired of grieving for humanity," she says, and the heat of her anger is in stark contrast to the prevailing mood of her previous work; she has closed off a chapter, died a little death to reemerge as a protest artist, not of understatement but of hot-hearted fury.

Tonight, she is restaging "Swanlights" for the Melbourne Festival, and I have bought a ticket; a cheap one, a last-minute release, which leaves me no time to think of reasons I should not go. I have forgotten what it feels like to sink into plush red seats and watch the lyrebird tails painted on the theater's curtains sway and ripple with the movement of the auditorium. The air is rich with evenings spent here as a child, when a friend of my parents passed ballet tickets to us; it feels like hushed silence, sitting on a pile of jumpers, eating scorched almonds out of tiny velvet bags.

For an hour and a half I am out of myself, out of time, back in my skin at last. Anohni herself is reassuringly present—a tall, solid figure in white, her long dark hair straggling on each side of her face. She looks like Cassandra, but her voice is not prophetic, only revelatory, in the sense of revealing to the audience what is already there, has always been there. A ripple of humor goes through the audience as the orchestra plays the opening bars of Beyoncé's "Crazy in Love," but stripped of its beat, it, too, is an elegy. The sparseness of its poetics, about the love that turns you to madness, and makes you plead to be saved from yourself, pulled out by the wrists, touches on something inside me that has been iced over for weeks.

It is a thumbprint on a sheet of frozen water. Anohni draws a breath and a tumble of words spills out, and she is no longer Cassandra—she is something like the plump sister in a '30s screwball comedy, giggling and flirting and leaving the fervor of transcendence behind. My mouth is full of salt and my breasts are full to brimming, and I have only so much time before I have to leave, but during the encore,

Boy George walks onto the stage. To an enthralled audience, he and Anohni sing,

> *I was so afraid of the night.*
> *You seemed to move through the places that I feared*
> *you lived inside my world so softly*
> *protected only by the kindness of your nature.*
>
> *You are my sister*
> *and I love you . . .*[16]

and I try not to measure the physical, visceral nature of their love for each other against the invisible relationship I have spun out of loneliness and need, an imaginary union with a woman who is doing everything that could be asked of her by simply standing in front of me, of us, and singing. It is the opposite of violence, and I don't yet know if I am ready for pressing, material love.

Still, I sit a long time in my seat once the concert is over. The curtains have closed; the lights are up again. I do not want to break the spell, but the room is emptying and my nipples are beginning to leak. Making sure I have my coat I leave the auditorium, find an accessible bathroom, then lean over the sink, one side of my bra unhooked as I lower my breast and press down above the areola. For a minute the sink fills with a milky blue light; then, stickily, I repeat the procedure, emptying myself out until the pangs of discomfort have passed.

SKYWHALE

THE WIND ON the hill is bitterly cold, with nothing between us and Hobart's icy seas. I huddle a little closer to Paulina for warmth. "Us" is her and me, and a gathered crowd of hundreds, waiting to see a hot-air balloon inflate— the Skywhale, the strange and compelling art balloon that has been bobbing around the country for weeks.

I've seen glimpses of the whale in press releases and on Twitter, where it spawns hashtags like tadpoles. In still images it is beautiful, somewhere between the ornate and the grotesque, bearing the hallmarks of designer Patricia Piccinini's sculptural practice. In person, it is an empty sack of industrial-strength nylon filling slowly with fire.

Breast upon delicate breast begins to undulate with heat. Children tear around gleefully, screeching, "It's weird!"

and "It's got *boobs!*" The figure emerges: a large, turtle-pated body, mottled in peachy pinks and grays, and ten enormous, drooping breasts.

Inflated, they are lovely—cupolas of hot air, rippling and then firming, their nipples grazing the lawn. Men in polar fleece dart forward past the barrier to take trompe l'oeil photos of themselves "holding" the nipples. *Wish you were here*, their gestures say.

I have come to Hobart for Dark Mofo, a festival celebrating the appetites of a gambling multimillionaire who has designed a contemporary art museum that will one day slide into the sea. I have come in a work capacity, but I have also come to stop breastfeeding.

I have been ready for months, but as soon as I try to disentangle myself from the baby, he goes on strike: solids, yes, but no liquid from any vessel other than me. I feed him before I go to work at the part-time job at a nonprofit I found after four months of desperate searching, and I come home at 6:30 p.m. precisely, for his evening feed. At 10:00 p.m. he wakes, and I feed him again.

This is the first time I've been so far from his stubborn, searching mouth. Mike is at home with a stash of bottles, some prefilled with frozen breast milk and others topped up with formula. He has lent me his army-issue green parka, soft and light like a sleeping bag. Walking along Hobart's quaint streets in my puffy coat and tight black jeans I think I must look like a cocktail olive, but I don't care.

I have only myself to look after. It is bliss.

What startles me is how little I have anticipated this: the lack of autonomy that comes from having a tiny child. Somehow when I was pregnant I managed to elide the breastfeeding into a narrative of separation: I would give birth, and we would be, with a small tinge of regret, no longer two synchronous rhythms in one shared body, but distinct: mother and child.

But there are hours: hours and hours of linking, because we aren't yet separate at all. In the hospital, I vomit from the Tramadol coursing through my IV, turning my head as Mike hastily takes the baby away, then reattaches him to the breast, the baby drawing sticky colostrum from my own body into his.

Owen is so tiny that I can *feel* the fluid traveling through his body. Pressed up against my skin, his little possum body convulses with happiness. He shits almost immediately after I feed him, mostly to be handed to Mike, who is full of love, while I sponge up any overflow that has sopped into my bra.

The day my milk comes in, home from the hospital, Mike stands behind me and pulls me into an embrace. I yelp; he jumps.

"Where can I hold you?" he asks anxiously.

The options are limited: my abdomen is still tender from layers of stitching after the birth, large staples forming a Joker mouth along the caesarean scar. My breasts feel like concrete. Mike touches one tentatively, and then whistles. He cannot believe how hard and large they are.

For the first few weeks, the baby and I are out of sync, with neither body knowing how to anticipate the needs of the other. I have borrowed a breast pump from a friend who has a toddler, a beautiful little girl who looks enormous next to Owen, but I am wary of wasting my still-chancy supply when Owen won't yet take a bottle. Inevitably, the minute I begin to pump, he wakes and begins to cry.

After a few months, things settle. The cluster-feeds die down into a steady rhythm, slowing the pace, giving us both room to breathe, and me time to marvel at this strange miracle of body knowledge. How can two such disparate entities get it so right? Now that he is feeding three-hourly, my body and his have become so attuned that my milk lets down one minute before he wakes from a nap, ravenous. I wonder what subconscious signals I am picking up, whether it is a trick of the mind or whether our bodies still *are* linked, so that mine receives advance warning through some etheric chain.

Two weeks after Owen's birth, Paulina swoops in in her old cream Skyline and takes me out for a coffee. We stay a little longer than I expect—it's a busy café—and race home to a screaming child. On the drive home, my breasts begin to ache.

I am hobbling, still, from the surgery. I hobble as fast as I can to the front gate, excusing my anxiety to Paulina.

"It's just that I have to be home to feed him."

"Just like a cow!"

She stops short.

"I'm so sorry."

"Forget it."

After a while, I stop sleeping at night. Insomnia settles in like a damp cloud. Everything feels a little bit damp—I find I cannot regulate my own temperature anymore. If I sleep, I wake drenched with sweat; I am going through two of Mike's old T-shirts every night. I have learned to place a towel on top of the sheet, to cut down on washing. We don't have a drier.

Mike and I have swapped sides of the bed; he is the crucial cog in the conveyor belt of keeping our child alive. Until my incision heals, I cannot pull myself up and over the side of the bed with any ease. Time in the army has taught Mike to sleep anywhere, immediately, a skill that I envy, and then, as the rot sets in, loathe him for. As soon as Owen stirs, Mike comes to, gently swings him over from the bassinet, then settles down to doze for forty-five minutes while I sit half propped up, wide-awake, icy and hot by turns, slowly being devoured.

Mike worries about me, and urges me to get out of the house. The rare times that I do, for gallery openings and

dinner parties, I learn to sneak off, to bend over the bathroom sink, contort myself, and express a small amount of
milk before my ducts give way and my bra is soaked through.
It doesn't occur to me to stop breastfeeding yet, though it is
beginning to exhaust me, burning through more energy
than I have to provide. The thought of getting out of a warm
bed at night, of preparing formula to the sounds of a shrieking child, of sterilizing bottle after bottle, seems more paralyzingly difficult than just whacking him on the breast.

In Hobart, I have booked a serviced apartment through one
of those deal websites that tells you the specifics of the hotel
but not the name. It has everything I need: it is central,
there is a king bed, there is a bath. I hate the cloistered
feeling of hotel rooms. Here, I have so much space.

I meet Paulina in Salamanca in the blinding white light
of the morning. She is delirious with art and novelty, and
also with pain. We walk through the small galleries that
have been set up around the docks, bumping into people
we vaguely recognize from Melbourne. They are easy to
pick. They are dressed more warmly than the Sydneysiders,
but are still visibly colder than locals.

Walking down the street I meet a friend's ex, who has
just had a baby with another woman. His long hair and
woolly jumper are bristling with static, enshrouding him
in a nimbus of glowing fuzz.

"How's the babe?" I ask.

"Oh, she's so good!" he says. "She sleeps really well and hardly ever cries."

He shuffles off into the sunlight. Paulina looks at me sideways. In the hard light, her face is blanched of color.

"What did it feel like when you were first pregnant?" she asks.

I try to think, to boil down the trepidation and uncertainty and tenderness and nausea and pain, and my body reads her body for subtext and clues.

"I'm only asking because my breasts are so sore. And I'm bleeding . . . a lot."

To the envy of the five- and six-year-olds in the crowd, we are allowed to skip the barricade as the Skywhale inflates. I am writing an article on the sculpture for a prestigious New York literary journal, which will eventually scrap the story for being "too Australian." Paulina is acting as my photographer. Our press credentials are golden tickets to the world of high-art ballooning.

The whale is supposed to fly gloriously over the duration of the nine-day festival, soaring above the nude swim and Winter Feast, but nearly every day a tweet has gone out apologizing for cancellations due to bad weather. This is the last day the balloon has a chance to fly, and it isn't able to really go up, simply inflate its capacity and bob gently, tethered to the ground.

One at a time we swing a leg over the side of the basket

and climb in. The sound of the flame is nearly deafening, and there is seemingly no logic as to when the balloon operator releases the jet: just a subtle touch, a glimmer of correspondence between man and whale that lets him know when a blast of heat is needed. It is difficult to interview him—this is the only time I've been able to wrangle. I ask him about his ten days as a performance artist, and Paulina takes photographs, and my audio recording reverberates with the sound of the blasts of flame.

The day is drawing later. We realize that we are on the point of the winter solstice, and madly, following some impulse of our own, Paulina and I link hands and race down the street to the ocean, greeting the shortest point in the year with a minute of reckless exultation, flushed from the run and salt-streaked from the spray that blows straight into our eyes.

I spend some of the next day in the core of the museum: MONA, the Museum of Old and New Art, dug into a heritage site accessible from the Hobart foreshore by ferry. I meet some of the curators for lunch, and, having skipped breakfast—I am sleeping long, uninterrupted stretches—become immediately tipsy from a prelunch glass of wine. It is fun to swan into the gallery's restaurant, to speak to brilliant curators and gallerists, try to find the sideways questions. I have missed doing this.

Half drunk, I spiral into the earth's core. First flight, now descent, but only equally as far—as the balloon was tethered, so the sandstone of the gallery's walls has been excavated and reinforced, insurance against a sudden collapse. It is still eerie to lose track of daylight. The museum has no real taxonomy; it showcases art of all genres indiscriminately, with iPods taking the place of information plaques. Each piece becomes unhitched from meaning, celebrating its founder's preoccupations.

There are breasts in here, too, and famously, a wall of porcelain vulvas. My favorite piece is Rafael Lozano-Hemmer's *Pulse Room*, an installation that measures the heart rate of each visitor and then flashes it through a series of bulbs, a different kind of conveyor belt, each heart light beating in and out of sync with the others. I have visited this work before, when I was pregnant, and imagined the tiny second heartbeat hidden deep in my own core.

Though I've brought the breast pump, I only have to duck back to the apartment a few times to use it. Either my body is frozen into submission, all nonessential processes retreating like bears into hibernation, or the physical distance—six hundred kilometers—is enough to fool me into thinking that this separation is real. In another city it is easy to forget my real life, to relax into a daily routine of sleep, coffee, art, dancing, booze. The truth is, I hardly think of my baby at all.

I suppose I should feel guilty about this, but I don't. I feel light on my feet, even blissful, in an echo of the way I remember life being before pregnancy stretched me out and weighed me down. My camera is heavy, but I am mercifully free of the nappy bag, extra nappies, wipes, change of clothes, bloody cumbersome pusher, and stash of apples and biscuits I usually carry. Stretched out in the large bed, I feel every muscle relax.

I check my Twitter feed intermittently, see how the Skywhale is doing on social media. There's a collective fondness for the sculpture that surprises me, a true engagement with this strange, engorged, mythical beast. I read that in Piccinini's created world, the breasts are functional: without wings to hold it aloft, the whale secretes a lighter-than-air gas from her breasts, propelling her upward.

The solstice is the shortest day of the year; most cultures associate it with some kind of rebirth or renewal. Image after image in my mental art history archive shows the coming of a spiritual savior with the dawn of the new year: Hors being resurrected as Koleda, Horus suckling at the breast of Isis, the infant Christ at Mary's breast, a one-way flow of nourishment from grown women to little boys.

I begin to fall in love with the whale and her maternal uplift. With ten pendulous teats she could nourish a city, but instead she has broken free of the demands of her invisible children and soars above them, benevolent, always moving upward. That idea of lightness stays with me for days.

On the closing Friday night of the festival, the tone is bacchanalian. I have to express, so come back to my little serviced unit. Paulina comes back with me and has a cup of tea curled up on the couch while I take a bath. The plan is to eat and then meet a photographer friend who knows the party planners, and immerse ourselves in the weird performativity of the festival evening.

The tea is necessary, particularly coming in from the dark, when our fingers are pink and barely working. I emerge from the bath even pinker, scrubbing myself down with a soft hotel towel and diving into my clothes before the chill can touch my skin. For the first time, I notice how truly wan Paulina is.

"Is it okay if I take a shower?" she asks.

"Of course," I say, and start chopping up dinner ingredients. They aren't fancy; I am living on the smell of an oily rag here, and can only cook what the tiny kitchenette will allow. Steam billows out of the bathroom and from the pot on the stove, tiny particles expanding to fill the room due to invisible, immutable laws.

A few minutes later, Paulina emerges wrapped in a towel, leaning dizzily against the wall. Her fine skin is blotched with pink, a fluorescent note of discord in her cheeks and across her chest.

"Jessica," she says quietly, "I think I'm having a miscarriage."

On a Friday night in a small strange town, there aren't many options for urgent care. I bundle Paulina into bed, then ring the front desk to ask if the apartments have an affiliated GP, someone who could come quietly and reassuringly—they don't. I have ideas about house calls that are probably twenty years out-of-date.

The receptionist suggests calling the paramedics when I tell her there might be a pregnancy involved. I pass my phone over when the connection is put through, and Paulina outlines her symptoms to them as I try not to hover. The paramedics decide they'd like to see her: they turn up ten minutes later, blocking in the rest of the guest parking, two lovely, competent women who chat with us about the festival and try to make Paulina feel at home.

In the end we wind up in the hospital; not the shrine to sex and death we were planning to visit that night, but not far from it. Paulina is hustled through triage by an officious nurse whose face I want to claw off for the implication that my friend is malingering. Who would be here by choice? The paramedics pull the nurse aside, their whisper too loud:

"We brought her in because we suspect a toxic abortion."

Paulina struggles to sit upright, indignantly:

"I haven't *had* an abortion!"

She is hustled off for a pregnancy test, which will later come back negative. The result is clear, and yet none of us can quite believe it. Paulina, the paramedics, me—we all have been menstruating for years, and we are all sure that something profoundly wrong is happening.

It is as though Paulina's pain is so hypnotically intense that her body has hallucinated a loss to explain it.

All the symptoms are there—the spasms, the nausea, the near-hemorrhage of blood—and collectively we cannot understand how this could be an ordinary process: *just* a period. The idea of a pain that *means* nothing; how can this make sense?

I wonder about the logic of emergency rooms. They seem almost affronted by the idea of sickness, and make no concession to it. The lights are overly bright, to hurt the eyes; the chairs are upright and painfully under-upholstered. A television set is almost always on, its volume somewhere on the border between hearing and not-hearing, so that ignoring it is an impossibility but seeking refuge in distraction is, too. In the distance we can hear the surreal soundscape of Ryoji Ikeda's *Spectra*, its white lights piercing the sky above the hill where yesterday we stood.

I send a text to our friend saying that we won't be meeting her. Paulina sends a text to her ex-boyfriend, outlining the situation. The clock crawls as the room fills with battered men, getting in early on their Friday night pub brawls; with vomiting children, infants crying incessantly. For the first time on hearing a crying child, my milk does not let down.

Paulina's cramps are coming in spasms and waves. She rests her clammy head on my shoulder, and I stroke her damp curls. Darling Pusia: the first person to know about my incipient child; my sister of choice, friend of ten years, former housemate; my dear, loud, Eastern European shouting companion. She tucks her knees up under her burnt-orange jumper, curling up against me like a child. The night ticks on, and I hold her, not to my breast, but to my heart.

CENTER STAGE, FIVE DANCES, AND OTHER DANCE ON-SCREEN

I HAVE BEEN watching a lot of ballet, on my laptop and on my phone. Every day, after delivering a toddling Owen to day care, having squandered the morning's energy on getting us both through the door, I make my way home and then back into bed, where no demands will be made of my body. The covers make a small stuffy cave, lit from within by the cool glow of the screen.

Over whatever semirespectable outfit I have cobbled together to face the outside world, I throw on a large shapeless jumper, often one of Mike's, and mismatched socks: one coming up to my knee and the other puddling around my ankle, too large but soft and woolly. These socks are called Explorers, which in some dim and dusty way, I know is funny.

I wrap myself in bed linen until there is no part of me that is not smothered and swaddled. It is safe to be entirely ensconced in blankets. On-screen, the dancers are almost bare, sheathed in thin leotards as they pirouette and chassé across the stage. I watch them, mesmerized, as the weight of my limbs and the weight of the blankets sink me into the softness of the mattress, the flannel sheets.

Raising your arms above your head, in ballet, is called a port de bras, a carriage of the arms. It corresponds to different foot positions depending on which school of dance you adhere to, but the arms are always graceful, supported from underneath, making strong lines that pull the body into alignment.

It is a movement that I call on when I try to hang the washing out. In the last few months, this has been an ungainly process, and sometimes impossible. I try to break *hanging out the washing* into a discrete choreography: gather two one-dollar coins—the machines will not take anything else—walk to the door, check for keys; pick up my basket, and walk it to the back of the apartment building, where two commercial washers locked in a shed are in a state of constantly breaking down.

Unlock the door, fumble my keys, load a washer; wait. Under my breath, I pray that I will not run into any of my neighbors, because I know I look like hell, and because I have no reserves for small talk right now. At any point the floodgates might open, and I am holding a breakdown at bay by sheer force of will.

The thought of speaking to anyone sends a ripple of nausea through me. Speech requires an effort I cannot make, not even for Mike, who soon will pick up the baby from day care, bring him home, and go about the nightly routine while I sit on the floor, attempting to force tears through a body that will not or cannot cry. When Owen is asleep, Mike will turn the lights down low for me, and sit next to me on the floor with a whisper of space between us, his steady breath easing the rapid flow of mine. He knows, even if he doesn't understand, how much the sound of the refrigerator hurts.

I watch ballet in fits and starts, in short bursts or embedded in various dance flicks; I cannot seem to manage anything else. The thing I watch most is *Center Stage*, the 2000 movie about aspiring ballerinas in New York, chasing their dreams. When Mike comes home and scoops me off the floor, it is this he often puts on.

In my illness I love this film wholeheartedly and without irony. I am the perfect passive vessel, and I let myself be overtaken by the fantasy of it. The film begins with a close-up of Jody, an aspiring ballerina, auditioning for the American Ballet Academy, lifting her arms at the barre, as a piano plays the opening bars of an *adage*. It is an image that is intimately familiar to anyone who has ever danced:

the barre, the rows of dancers, the instructor counting out beats in soft, steady streams of French, and it transports me back immediately to a time when I knew this in my own body.

The lighting is soft and clean, lingering on the room's various but synchronous figures; you can almost smell the rosin, and feel the warmth of bodies as they relax and stretch. The plot is simple, for a brain that is exhausted past coherence. As in ballet itself, there is virtually no subtext: the action is purely textual, each scene propelling itself into the next, which is what I need right now—for something to appear exactly as it is.

Although much of the narrative padding of the film is in its love triangle, it is really about a dancer's crisis of confidence. When we meet Jody, her physique is imperfect, her technique is lagging; as classes begin, she starts to question whether she should attempt to dance ballet at all. Despite solitary late-night rehearsals, she falls behind; she sleeps with choreographer Cooper, is cast in his workshop piece, and then discovers that she is not even close to the only woman he is seeing. She is young, nervy, naive, a wreck; but there is something *there*, waiting to be discovered.

After she is humiliated by Cooper in a rehearsal, Jodie storms out in tears, followed by sweet love interest Charlie. He calms her down and tells her that her volatility is an asset, that it fuels her interpretive range, that she was accepted into the academy for this intangible artistry, which she does not know how to trust.

"Whatever you feel," he says, "just dance it."

Oh God, it's so cheesy and mawkish, but my heart goes out again and again, watching Jody wipe her face, walk back in, and then, through some process of alchemy, launch into a sequence of steps that supports and transforms her. There is something in my own body that flows out to meet the screen, something almost like catharsis, which lifts the weight in my limbs, if only for a minute at a time.

I am astonished to learn later that there's a name for this, the deeply regenerative feeling of watching somebody else dance, even when your own body is sluggish and sick and impossible to navigate. It is known in dance movement therapy as *kinesthetic empathy*: an innate response of the body to movement in the bodies of others.

Theodore Lipps hypothesised this in the nineteenth century with the concept of *Einfühlung*, an "inner mimesis," but science now knows it to be true; the 1996 discovery of the mirror neuron confirmed that the brain doesn't just store information about the movements of others, but interiorly mimics it, sending shock waves of phantom experience through our bodies in the hopes that they might anticipate the real thing.

The dance critic John Martin, whose appointment at *The New York Times* saw dance examined critically in its own right as a modernist form, posited this in 1936, arguing that movement should be divorced from the narrative constraints of the story ballet and extend itself in pure form to an audience that is active, rather than passive. He writes:

> We shall cease to be mere spectators and become participants in the movement that is presented to us, and though to all outward appearances we shall be sitting quietly in our chairs, we shall nevertheless be dancing synthetically with all our musculature. Naturally these motor responses are registered by our movement-sense receptors, and awaken appropriate emotional associations akin to those which have animated the dancer in the first place. It is the dancer's whole function to lead us into imitating his actions with our faculty for inner mimicry in order that we may experience his feelings.[1]

In Martin's schema, emotion can be transferred from one being to another through a kind of psychic synthesis of performer and audience. As modern critics have written, this is naive; it disclaims cultural difference, subjectivity, difference in physical ability and disability, as well as myriad other sociohistorical factors. (How does someone without a leg "experience" an arabesque? How do those with neurological impairments "mirror" gesture?)

But there's something compelling about the purity of his idea. In asking the watcher to imagine herself as the dancing body, and rise to match its emotional intent, Martin asks the watcher to become imaginatively more flexible, limber, elevated to the level of a professional. It lifts us, even fleetingly, from our stodgy and broken bodies into a—fictitious—realm, where a universal language of gesture and emotion is not only possible, but natural.

This empathy isn't restricted to the experience of watching live dance. There is a kinesthetic relationship inherent in moviegoing that supports the resonance of the series of movements in *Center Stage*, or *The Red Shoes*, or *Dance Academy*, which I watch again and again; the fourth wall lifts like a red curtain, leaving nothing between the dancing body and the watching one, per Martin's notion.

Some of these movements have shaken their way through my body; as a child I took ballet classes, like so many other young girls, long-limbed, gangly, and with feet too highly arched—and yet I was serene and content in the ignorance of my own shortcomings. The physical echo of these classes stays with me, somewhere. I feel it as a pang when Owen sits up, perfectly straight-backed, his feet tucked neatly beneath him; when Mike comes in from a run, his face pink with exertion and his thigh muscles pulsing and contracting as he begins to cool down.

And I feel it in my dreams. At night, I think often that I am dancing, in the same way that in dreams I can perfectly speak French, and I don't know if it is a synthesis of all that I have learned, pulled together perfectly in my subconscious, or simply a trick of the mind. In sleep, I feel my legs extend far past the arabesques of my childhood; I feel my footwork tidy and brisk as my arms raise, and my too-long toes miraculously bear the weight of my legs and hips, pelvis sturdy, as I rise up on phantom pointe. Always I wake with a sense of loss. The exhilaration slips away, and I realize that this body that has moved so recklessly and gracefully through my dreams does not exist in fact.

As I watch others dance, and these mirror neurons fire, other neurons falter. My brain's wells of serotonin and nor-epinephrine are running dry. Quietly, as I sleep, my body is overtaken by a protective sluggishness that conserves energy, cuts its expenditure down to the barest necessary functions. When I wake, it is often with a low thrum along my bones, which travels from humerus to scapula, making my shoulders feel battered. If I feel this ache, I know it will be a hard day.

It still baffles me to a degree that this illness, experienced to the fullness of its logic, is characterized as "mental" when it is so punishingly physical, as though the brain isn't a part of the body, cherished and integrated; or as though any illness originated in the brain will be contained there, and not leak and spill and overflow it.

I have only had a general anesthetic once, but I remember vividly the feeling of blankness rushing up my arm and to my mind. Now it feels as though the numbness is traveling in the other direction. Depression seems to be composed of lack: anhedonia, aphasia, insomnia, all a-words, existing *outside*, like atheism exists outside, and is banished from, the idea of the church. This body, I have been told, is a temple, but slowly I am becoming excommunicated from myself.

As illness trickles down, my sense of perception is thrown out, so that it constantly seems as though doorframes aren't where I left them, and cups of tea overflow from juddering hands. Lifting my arms above my shoulders to dress becomes difficult, as does bending over to tie my shoelaces. Sitting on the edge of the bed, my feet seem unfathomably far away, as do memories and words and meanings; Mike often has to repeat things twice, three times, before I understand what it is he is trying to say.

Depression and anxiety are twins; they follow each other around. When the anxiety flares up, the sluggishness is shot through with hyperarousal—a raw exposing of all the senses to one's surroundings. Lights become far too bright, sounds overwhelmingly loud, and my skin feels stretched so thin as to bruise at the softest touch. The detergent aisle is the first site of exile, rebuffing me even if I reach it; the various powders and soaps are too strong and chemical. Then it is fluorescence, the white noise, the whir of central air, the squeak of shoes on linoleum. I walk to the edge of the supermarket and then stand there paralyzed, unable to go in.

In this state of hyperarousal, pain tolerance is also lowered. Things hurt more. The startle reflex is exaggerated; I jump at the sound of cats, of car doors, and my son, toddling into the bedroom to grab me for a game. It feels like a testament to my love for him that I do not shriek, but let him clamber over me, hating it and him and the world as my mood plummets swiftly, too quick and dangerous for him to catch. I scrutinize myself for proofs of love, and they always seem to be in the not-doing, negative proofs; not shrieking, not breaking, not passing my anger on into his tiny form.

When I am sick, I am slow, and heavy, and hateful, almost physically and certainly psychically debilitated. I cannot speak and I cannot scream, but I can resonate like a cello string, turn my eyes from the hard outside world toward the structured, choreographed, distant one, where dance remembered in the body and seen on-screen keeps some inarticulable part of me tethered to the earth. *Bodies*, this dancing seems to say. *People feel love in their bodies.*

The dance film is most often divided into two parts, rehearsal and performance, the tension of one informing the release of the other. *Center Stage* ends with a contemporary ballet performed in its entirety and mirroring almost everything that has happened in the film preceding it— the opening of the ballet echoes the opening of the film, and it recapitulates the film's love triangle, right down to Cooper driving his motorcycle across the stage.

The sequence of steps that Jodie transforms radiantly through her tears in the film's rehearsal scene is seen again, repeated as a passage in this larger production, one that celebrates her extremely minor physical imperfections and ends with her triumphantly spinning in a series of fouetté turns, giddy with joy in her own artistry. In part, *Center Stage* is such a perfect sick-day film because of this pattern of rehearsal/anguish giving way to performance/catharsis; there is a narrative predictability that impels feel-good-ness—a mirror-twin of feeling good.

I don't want to think about the ongoingness of pain, and although the film makes a feature of early shots of dancers' feet, bruised and scraped, and watches them rehearse lonely passages in classrooms late at night, its ending puts Jodie's anguish and indecision behind her forever. She is a principal now, a founding member of a new company; her hard work has paid off, her prince has come. I don't want to think of her damaging her ligaments, or plunging her bruised feet into a bucket of ice, because I want to believe in the fairy tale. I want to believe that hard work will give way to lyrical motion; that the thing underscoring this gestural beauty is not damaging, grueling effort, but exhilaration and flight.

I do not watch any full-length story ballets, I realize, in part because I am becoming addicted to this pattern of rehearsal and performance, effort and release. It is not hard to find a *Giselle* or a *Rite of Spring* online, but their seamlessness turns me away. Instead, I watch the behind-the-scenes featurettes that the Australian and London and New York City Ballets turn out almost weekly, little movies about dancers who are phenomenally gifted, but warm and funny and real.

I download Alan Brown's *Five Dances*, almost a complete inversion of *Center Stage*, a low-key documentary-style indie film in which the dances of the title are woven through the film as completed works. Its five characters are four dancers and a choreographer, rehearsing and creating a new piece. The dances are both polished artifacts, the earned outcomes of physical hard work, and dreamlike interpolations of the choreography as it is presented in rehearsal: they refract and reflect the four key characters' emotional states. They are beautiful.

The choreography, attributed in-film to fractious choreographer Anthony, is by Jonah Bokaer, who danced with the Merce Cunningham Dance Company; Cunningham is cited in the film, and it is clear that this choreography is explicitly informed by Martin's and Cunningham's ideas of dance as direct communication, not through narrative, but through movement. The film is shot through with the vocabulary of "shapes" and "channels," which echo Martin's idea of "paths," or traces left by dance in the body of both the dancer and the spectator.

As I begin to try various drugs and cognitive therapies, rechoreographing the neural pathways of my brain, I try also to refute my physical inertness. I start to teach myself the vocabulary of choreography; there is something about its simplicity and suppleness that, as Cunningham says, bypasses language to rattle around the body itself. As the film is broken up—rehearsal/performance, rehearsal/performance—I find myself noticing the resonances flowing both ways; choreography and performance are symbiotic, they feed each other.

I realize, too, that what I have been doing in choreographing my laundry is actually called "marking." Dancers don't always rehearse to the full extent the performance requires; it would expend too much energy, cost too much. Instead, they extend their hands and feet out in soft motions, small maquettes of the gesture that is soon to be reproduced in full. I cannot get to a full port de bras yet, but I am marking it, and thus keeping it in my body for the day I have the strength to wring and hang out my cold, sodden sheets.

What I am also marking is time. I know this is an expression—*marking time*—but I am constantly reassured by the twinned, pinned-together facts of space and time that dance so calmly unfolds. In the mountain of my piled-linen bed, a minute can last an hour or a day. Choreography regulates time, it enfolds it; I am constantly amazed by the quickness, the almost devastating quickness of ballet; a series of gestures pass in an eight-count bar that would take me hours to accomplish.

Everything happens on the count, everything unfurls. As my physical endurance begins to improve, I start thinking seriously about moving again, beyond the hesitant, incentive-based walks I am able to take with the assistance of antidepressants—little missions, like getting Owen to day care, going to the library, leaving the house to get a coffee. At first I need an incentive, a bribe. Motion for its own sake makes me feel too tentative, too wobbly, but I begin to get steadier on my feet.

After a few months, I sign up for a conditioning class based on ballet movement; I need small warmings of the muscle, soft extensions, to guide me back into physical movement, and I am still worried about the too-fast pace of my heartbeat, my too-shallow breath.

All these months of depression have stripped away what little muscle tone I once had, leaving me feeling airless and unsupported. I sketch my pointed toes out in experimental, small circles, trying to remember the feeling of strong weight in my legs making these shapes precise and clean.

As the class begins, with breathing and stretches, I try to get my body to relax. Nobody claps; there is no pianist here, simply a group of adult women, making time in their day to lift, bend, extend, curve, and release. Heat flows through my chest and shoulders as they slowly open out, releasing more tension than I am aware of carrying. My arms do not stretch very far, but I am pleased that they can open at all.

For the duration of the warm-up and isometric exercises I keep up, but when the pliés begin, and I compare my body to other bodies, it is clear that I am far, far behind in form. Like Jodie in *Center Stage*, my turnout is poor; where for her, imprecision means a couple of degrees from perfection, my hips will only turn out to a right angle, throwing my knees far out in front of what should be a two-dimensional plane.

But the heat searing my inner thighs as I try to force them outward is a good heat, I think. It is agony, but after months of lying frozen and inert, it is welcome.

I want to keep the classes up, but they are too expensive. Months pass. I put my hand on the windowsill and pretend it is the barre, trying to sink gracefully, trying to push myself past the point of exertion in which I want to simply give up. The vocabulary of self-care emphasizes gentleness, knowing one's bounds, and I grapple with the paradox that to make any forward motion I will need to push *through* these bounds; I wish my skin were a chrysalis.

It is becoming easier to practice, though, to maintain my breath, to loosen my joints. I sit in the winter sunshine with Mike, leaning against him at the park while Owen scurries around the playground and practices his own new skills: climbing a chain-link ladder, balancing on a very low beam. Owen demands my presence, and uses my hands as an extension of his own body; it is what I am there for, to be braced against. To an extent, we engage in a constant pas de deux: our bodies move in response to the other's needs, and when I lift him, his feet push off the ground; I know the sound of his breath intimately, but it is overwhelmingly an unequal partnership.

I am finding a way back to my body and I am finding a way back to Mike's body, but it is difficult. Where I can dredge up and cajole energy for Owen, it still leaves me depleted; Mike knows that the physical love and tenderness

I show to Owen is for him as well, but I am aware of the blank weight between us that is the absence of touch. I wonder how much of my fantasy about dance is a fantasy of touching again, about wanting and wanting to be fit for the emotional weight of touching, of movement, of sensory engagement that can bear the forces of intimacy and sensuality as well as grace and speed.

I watch the dancers on-screen, so casual in their own bodies, in Jody Lee Lipes's *Ballet 422*. In this film there is some rehearsal, barely any performance. The camera follows Justin Peck, at the age of twenty-five, as he choreographs a new work for the New York City Ballet. The film is broken into the percussive rhythms of iteration, of movement of all kinds: of an elegant hand cutting out costumes, and a mouth chewing gum; of a conductor elaborating a choreography of his own; of dancers sewing shoes, and lighting designers calling out an incomprehensible liturgy of spot- and down-light marks.

It takes patience to watch; I can only sit still, endure the film's deliberate slowness, when I am more or less in my own skin again. Still, when I *am* able to watch it I sink into it; it is easy to inhabit this world. I expect to feel a kind of reactionary envy of Peck, who is a genuine wunderkind, but instead something stirs in unlikely allegiance. "I'm not a very good dancer," he says in an interview when asked about his flaws; good enough to make the corps de ballet, eventually soloist, but not marked with the fierce burning talent of the principals in his company.

And yet there is something *in* him that I know so well;

an urge to express movement beyond what his body is capable of, in a way that is more beautiful, more precise than he can ever himself achieve. It is amazing to watch him, mumbling and almost paralyzingly inarticulate, somehow convey his vision; to pull the lights and costumes and music together into something discrete and whole and inextricably his. To express it, I have to express it in the language of movement itself; I am moved, and I am touched.

When the next summer has passed, and the nights are getting cooler, and I am at least shakily certain of my own ability to exert control over my body, Paulina and her friend Whil and I take an impromptu hiking trip. I call it "hiking," but for me it is really just brisk walking, which is still a cause for celebration. Whil has brought his own little tent, but the first night is so chilly that we all pile into Paulina's big one, bought cheap and cheaply made. In the morning we find condensation forming inside the fly, but in the evening, snuggled together on layers of blankets and towels and buried under unzipped sleeping bags, it is cozy, almost comfortably warm.

We climb to the top of the hill, and Whil goes off to clamber some more, while Paulina and I lie like snakes in the sun. I take off my bra and stuff my T-shirt between the patch of rock we are lazing on and my naked skin, feeling thin heat hit every muscle in my torso. There is a breeze, but it is invigorating. When Whil returns I pull my top back on, and we cobble together makeshift sandwiches, but by the end of the day we are all skinny-dipping in the freezing river, rinsing off our filthy feet and hands as the occasional car wends around the curves in the road above.

Whil has just finished a show in which he has played various animals. Standing in a field of native grass, he suddenly arches his back and arms, and for a second he is not Whil but a looming black swan. The impression lasts for a few beats, and then we continue on, using our arms and legs and core muscles in utilitarian, human ways.

It is glorious, glorious motion. My well body fills me with an exultation that is not entirely uncoupled from guilt and shame. And I know I have not been alone in my fantasies, but still: I have fantasized about being hit by a car; I have fantasized about breaking my leg; about being made immobile, absolved of worry; I have played out anxieties on the surfaces of and within my skin.

Most of all, at the beginning of depressive episodes when everything is still internal, I have wished that my illness were not invisible; that depression manifested as a series of scars, or extra fingernails growing up my arms. I have envied, sickly, the people I have known who were anorexic or bulimic, for the way in which their illnesses have been legitimated and recognized, *visible*, while mine manifested only as a lack.

And yet I know how twisted the logic of this is. There is fleeting satisfaction that comes from physical pain, from inertia, but it is swamped by the frustrations and irritations and sheer exhaustion of ongoing unwellness. When I lean against Owen's pusher, roughly the size of a wheelchair,

I am acutely aware of the spaces it cannot access; that my limbs—which I cannot raise above my head some days and that Mike swathes in jumpers and pants, in the same way he helped me tie my shoes when I was voluminously pregnant—that these limbs still hold the germs of their ability, are only temporarily sluggish and slow.

When I am well, the body wants to forget; it is so eager to stretch and bend, to repress any residual traces of illness. It is a necessary mechanism for healing, I suppose, but it is a cruel one. One of the dance pieces I come back to, again and again, is Lucy Guerin's *Untrained*, in which untrained dancers mimic onstage the leaps and steps of professionals. It could be played for laughs, but it is immensely touching seeing these men approach new physical challenges, reaching for the grace of the dancers they are mimicking, or simply searching for the possibility of a movement they have never before accomplished.

Illness and health, movement and inertia; they are not dialectically opposed, but constantly approaching and retreating from one another, overlaying each other, coexisting. My brain, when tired and slow, wants the release of an easy catharsis, but my body knows that life is in the iteration; how many times have we turned off the lights together, turned a key in the lock, made soup? We are partners, my body and I.

When I am well, I tell myself—not just neutrally "not unwell," but intellectually fleet and stable and coherent and energetic, if I ever am again—I will cast off the teen dance flicks and look further. Dance about corporeality, about the ill and unwell body, is of course prolific. But at the present I cannot bring myself to watch *Still/Here*, Bill T. Jones's dance about people with terminal illness, much as I cannot encounter Tatsumi Hijikata's brutally grotesque *butoh*. I cannot bring myself to watch the choreography of Meg Stuart, who asks her dancers to return again and again to the site of their first encounter with a specific choreography, mimicking their mistakes exactly.

These things are too close to the body, to my body, to my sense of sinking rapidly. When I am at my worst, I want only to be buffeted by the narrative simplicity, the fluff, of a film such as *Center Stage*; it balances out the darkness. It is only when I am healthy that I can stand the complexity and mess and heartache of reality. Perhaps, in this sense, illness and health form a dialectic after all.

In the meantime, Paulina takes me to see Whil's new show at the Abbotsford Convent. It is nominally about Catholicism, and there are theatrical elements that do not work for me, but the dance itself is superb. Untrained, Whil's lines are idiosyncratic, reaching, not emulating the verticality of ballet, but shaky and curved. His costume is all white, a jeweled top and a pair of quilted culottes, and as he shuffles forward with his arms grasped above his head he reminds me of that swan again; his silhouette, for a second, takes on the traditional contours of men's costuming in *Swan Lake*, and he is both more and less than human. From my seat a hand span away, I see his sweat, I hear his breath, and for a minute, the space between us is so charged as to nearly be no space at all.

ALTERED NIGHT

IN KATHMANDU, HELEN and I spend a lot of time on the rooftop, playing backgammon. We have come to visit during a lull in Nepal's strange and tense political season; there is a stalemate between the Maoist rebels in the countryside and the army camped in the cities, and the result is a kind of peace, an openness to the circulation of foreign bodies that is tied to a needed circulation of money. I am sure that Helen and I have some pretensions about being travelers and not tourists, but that is what we are; young, still in our teens, with strong teeth and bones, and our passports in the pockets of our borrowed backpacks.

Helen has been to India and Nepal before; I have not. It is my first time traveling independently, and I am heady with the freedom of it. For the first two days we wander, shaking off our jet lag, and pick up trinkets in various shops, try on earrings, look at textiles. Then our freedom is curtailed—the government has called for a daylong curfew, with no one allowed to leave their homes, in order to stymie a prodemocracy demonstration that is supposed to take place in Durbar Square. The enforced stillness confines us to our beds, lazy and reading, until we need fresh air and emerge onto the roof.

I am not used to schooling myself to stillness. Back home, I have been a whirlwind: going to gallery openings, going to uni, working in a deli to save up for the trip. I am living at home still, so each fortnight a few hundred dollars—the fruit of hours spent handling olives and cheese and meat—comes into my account and does not go out again on rent or bills. I am a vegetarian, but our boss at the deli does not believe in wearing gloves. It is cleaner, he insists, to scrub your bare hands between serving each customer, but still my hands are larded at the end of each shift with six hours' worth of fat and salt. When I get home the dog goes berserk, smelling the protein on me, thinking that I have brought him a treat.

I am conscious of how I smell when I go straight from the deli to uni. Even with a change of clothes, the odor of fat clings to me; it seems to get into my hair, the way cigarette smoke does until bars are declared smoke-free. Toward Christmas, my job is to prepare hams out the back of the shop, peeling their top fat back and scoring the flesh into diamonds, which are studded with cloves, and smeared with orange marmalade and juice before we pile them into the oven. The only part of this I enjoy is the peppery, fresh scent of cloves.

In Nepal, the question of food is easy; vegetarianism is not strange. We sit in a little restaurant called the Momo Cave, eating dumplings and drinking endless cups of tea. By the time the curfew is relaxed, the stillness has taken hold, and we dawdle; I want to linger on all sensations, luxuriate in books, sleep in, let warm milk coat my mouth and tongue. Most of all, I want to look at everything, and try to discipline myself not to stare.

I have read Edward Said in Art History and am trying to practice an ethical aesthetic consumption, but the pleasures of novelty are so tantalizing. I look and look at the flags of laundry fluttering out across Kathmandu's rooftop gardens, which make a map of color in the air. There is something about the light in the Northern Hemisphere that makes the sky seem closer, flattening the world a little, but drawing it nearer. I look at the stray dogs slinking around the roads, the men wandering around selling individual clove cigarettes. Helen and I sit on the roof of our hotel and talk into the evening, and I watch the blond of her hair turn rosy with the setting sun.

When my hand is not occupied with backgammon pieces, it often moves across the page, scrawling down small, incomprehensible notes. I take a camera with me, but don't photograph often, feeling bashful about it. Instead, I keep a notebook, writing impressions, and half-overheard conversations, and fragments of poetry. The camera and the book serve the same purpose; I have been looking forward to the experience of traveling, but it turns out that what I want from this experience is to mediate it; to fix it immediately, to layer something of myself on it, or it on me. As much as I try simply to *be*, my brain keeps wanting, greedily, to do.

With Helen I don't have to explain this. From the earliest days of our friendship, as very young children, what has always joined us is our mutual compulsion to make things; we are most comfortable in the art room at school. At each other's houses, our mothers encourage our relentless production. From our hands come papier-mâché, and hand-painted pillows sewn with wonky seams; flowers pressed in the pages of books, pom-poms, cross-stitch, and slightly grubby Fimo. Each thing we treasure for a short while, and then move on from, as our skills become greater and our visions more ambitious.

In photos of the two of us we hang upside down on gates, go yabbying, jump over creeks, but often our faces are twinned as we bend over our sketchbooks; our expressions reflect the intense satisfaction that total concentration on creating something provides.

It's a concentration that appears on Owen's little face, when he strings beads along a piece of thread or adds ten legs to a drawing of an elephant. Seen from the outside, it is just as compelling, and just as utterly mysterious.

In terms of developing skills, his work makes sense— at a base level, stringing beads develops his fine motor skills, spatial awareness, and hand-eye coordination—but what remains cryptic to me is the need and desire to make it *art*; he could learn these skills counting dried beans into a mixing bowl, which he also enjoys, but quickly the game develops to include specific colors and patterns, little rituals. I clip the end of the piece of thread with a tiny peg, to keep the larger beads from slipping off the end, and he demands a little peg every time we play.

The thread, too, has to be purple—a piece of lilac embroidery floss from a jar of flosses bought at a garage sale. The needle he threads his beads over must be my curved haberdashery needle. The things he threads grow tinier and tinier, and I marvel at the precision of his small hands; at three, he is capable of threading the needle through the tiny eyes of very little buttons, something I struggle to do without my glasses. At a certain point, determined by him, the string is resolutely done, and the thing that he has made is always called "A Rainbow Snake," to be played with, admired, undone, and then made again.

Siri Hustvedt, in her essay "Embodied Visions," points out that it is only humans who seem to have a drive toward the creation of art, despite the tales of painting elephants and monkeys, and pins this drive directly to the development of subjectivity, specifically reflective self-consciousness. "All animals have drives," she writes, "most notably to survive, but making art is not about survival, despite the fact that many artists feel that if they couldn't do their work, their lives would lose meaning."[1]

What, then, *is* making art all about? Hustvedt suggests

that it is, in some forms, an extended variance on imaginative play, again unique to humans and crucial to impel the ability to "see" and conceptualize the self as a double figure—one in the realm of physicality, one in fantasy or trance; explaining the prereflective (subconscious) awareness she feels when sitting in a chair, she adds:

> But let us say that while I am in the same chair I
> get it into my head to do a self-portrait of myself
> in the chair, and I fetch a pencil, paper, and a
> mirror so I can see myself and begin to draw.
> The idea expressed in the words—*I'll draw
> me*—entails a splitting of myself into both subject
> and object, and this self-reflective distance is an
> essentially human adventure.

I like this focus on art as both embodied and psychic, and the essay is an excellent one, as are, in fact, all of her writings on art. But the fact that art is perhaps essential, as a form of play, to the development of human subjectivity doesn't adequately explain why as subjectivity becomes more complex, the creation of art becomes more difficult; why for some of us, interior visions can be matched by dexterity and skill, and why the rest of us shift from an experience of art that is about *making* to one that is about *looking*.

It's a trick question in a way, given Hustvedt's focus on the art act as one of mirroring—as a crucial player in the creation of mirror neurons, and the positing of both an *I* and a *you*. If art is a mirror, and presupposes a voyeur who can also be ourselves, then making and looking become somehow a synonymous act.

By the time we are at university, Helen and I have made the transition to scrutiny. I haven't seen her in years—I got put up a year level, she went to a different school—but almost immediately we are by each other's sides, both of us taken up with classes in art history. We meet for coffee outside the Elisabeth Murdoch building, which houses the art library and a large lecture theater, and chat in a mixture of extremely poor French and Japanese. Unconsciously, we are falling into a childhood secret language. It is like falling in love. It *is* falling in love. When she suggests that we save up and go backpacking around India and Nepal together, I do not hesitate to say yes.

In Delhi, we stop off for a few days and spend our time drinking coffee in a little café that is predominantly frequented by Japanese tourists. We make friends with a Japanese photographer and bum around with him, not wanting to rush, simply sitting and soaking everything up. We do make our way to the gallery, though, which is staging a major retrospective of the works of Amrita Sher-Gil, an artist I haven't heard of until now.

The room is whitewashed for this show; I am struck by the vividness of color emanating from the paintings. At first, I feel the same feelings that stir my gut when I look at a reproduction of Gauguin, but these paintings are clearly different: they are painted more compassionately, with a feminist gaze; I do not have to ask myself, as I ask about Gauguin, what the *intention* was in choosing any particular model. The works span just over a decade, and become more deliberately naive, or abstracted, as time passes.

I am startled, though, to find the line of my own profile in a self-portrait from 1931. Sher-Gil sits, shoulder slumped forward, peering off to the right of the frame, a yellow beret perched upon her head. It turns out that Sher-Gil's mother, like my father, was a Hungarian Jew; Amrita spent her childhood in Budapest, absorbing the tones and techniques of its painters, so the resemblance is not totally impossible, though the similarities fade as I look at it more closely. I peer at this painting for a long time, trying to unravel the mystery of how I can appear in a ghost form of line before I am born and meet myself later, halfway around the world.

Back home, I move out to a share house with Paulina, and go about the work of trying to become a writer. I switch from art history to creative writing, and volunteer at a youth literary organization, sitting on the board and learning about governance. When I land a job editing the student union's newspaper, I am overjoyed; the fact that the wage comes in well below the poverty line doesn't faze me. It is more money than I have ever earned at the deli, or waitressing, and it is still cheap to live in the inner city.

The fact that I have never experienced true poverty

inures me; this is merely "being broke," a chronic condition for those of us in the arts. Through a lens of adventure, it can seem romantic. Paulina and I visit the markets in the afternoon and buy boxes of squashy tomatoes, simmering them down into sauce, and eat stone fruit off our trees. Helen has been volunteering at an independent gallery for years, and often trades a catalog essay for a painting or a sculpture, so that the walls of her bedroom are increasingly precious in value. We both find ways to save money where we can.

"What exactly is the basic shape of this haircut?" I ask, considering Helen's face reflected back at me in the mirror, her shoulders draped in a towel.

"The basic shape of this haircut, I would say, is a pyramid," she replies, passing me the scissors.

When things become materially difficult, I remind myself that I have chosen to do this, that living month by month as a freelancer is a choice. After a few years, the romance has worn off, and I begin to dread winter, not just for the damp rising through the weatherboard walls of my house, but for the tonsillitis I inevitably get and the dent it puts in my ability to work. When I get a urinary tract infection for the third time in two months, I go to the sexual health clinic and not the doctor at university, because even though both bulk-bill, the sexual health clinic often gives out free antibiotics.

Helen has been offered a semester at Georgetown, and we send each other long emails after she leaves. I get my hair cropped short at the hairdressing academy, spending an afternoon as a hair model for a free cut, and send her a photo. When the loneliness and the cold and the sense of always being a bill payment behind becomes too much, I take heart from Ruth Park and D'Arcy Niland, determined to make their livings as writers during the Second World War, working frenetically, never losing faith, eventually honing their distinctive voices through commitment to their craft. It is a privilege, I think, to be able to commit yourself to an art—any art—and this is what I tell myself as I churn out terrible poems, the sheets of my bed so cold they are damp. If things get really bad, I can always go to my parents' house for dinner.

What strikes me about these years, when I try to recall them now, is how indistinct they seem. The energy and the momentum, underwritten by anxiety, smudges each day into the next. Sometimes there isn't sleep to break the hours into discrete, named chunks; in these weeks, I know that depression is coming for me, and work myself into even more of a frenzy, before the lassitude pulls me under.

The pace that I keep up, and that Helen keeps up, is expected; in fact, it is required. Publishing, curatorial practice—both are "glamour" industries, where the self-evident good of the work is supposed to make up for low pay, few industrial protections, plenty of unpaid overtime. It is not just that it *is* a privilege to do the work; the work itself requires privilege, cultural capital, mobility.

Years seem to go by in a blur of gallery openings, magazine launches, funding crises. There is Helen, blond head gleaming, looking like a pile of sacks in her artfully draped gallery gear; there am I, sitting at the kitchen table at three a.m., reading short-story submissions as moths batter themselves against the window. Helen picks up tutoring shifts; I get more and more freelance work. As when we were children, we have barely finished one thing when a vision of another emerges, something bigger, more compellingly urgent.

It is exciting to feel as though we are being midwives to other people's work; this is what editing and curatorship have in common. As the money in both of our professions gets tighter, and our jobs seem to encompass more and more, we dig in our heels; the closing ranks of bigger institutions makes it seem more crucial to produce work we believe in, to support artists we feel will make some kind of difference to the cultural landscape.

I see, but do not want to acknowledge, older women vanishing over the horizon. I hold to Ruth Park, writing with five small children, and Rumer Godden, waking at four a.m. so that she could write before the babies were up. I can already feel other demands beginning to compete with the relentless need for work—I have almost taken Saint Benedict's words, "Work is prayer," as my motto—and wish I had a mentor, someone older than me, more balanced, with a ten-year glimpse into the future.

Instead, I turn to the women I know, who more and more prop one another up. It is a remarkable group, and I am lucky to be part of it: this ever-shifting crowd of writers and artists who listen, share, support. Mostly I crash on Helen's floor, and she on mine, and together we are quiet, relaxed; "Jessie, my gal!" she cries, hugging me loosely, without a trace of makeup and swathed in her big red jumper. There is a divine normalcy in her company, and familiarity, closeness. It is a tonic, to draw from twenty years of offhand conversations.

Helen is the person I tell when I lose my virginity, and when I fall in and out of love, and she is the person I ask to be my witness when I elope to the registry office with Mike. The night beforehand, Mike goes out for a beer with his witness, Mark, and I go a little frenetic alone in the house by myself, and decide to get my eyebrows waxed. My waxer isn't in, so I have my brows threaded instead, by a woman who misunderstands my directions and leaves me feeling like I have no eyebrows at all.

I text Helen, wailing, and turn up on her doorstep.

"Oh, they're not so bad!" she says, giving me a straight Helen look. "Don't be silly. Come in, I have some really disgusting red wine."

We sit on the floor and I begin to relax. Helen's share house is a run-down terrace in Fitzroy, the walls a salmon pink that is dated but which I love. They are lined with paintings and hung with bits of sculpture, her collection having grown. I am always particularly drawn to a small group of paintings by her housemate Clare's boyfriend,

Sean, a series of small square collages that have been painted over in vibrant tones.

"Did you bring a bit of that fabric?" Helen asks.

She means a scrap from my wedding dress, the shoulder pads of which I have removed. Mike and I have barely scraped up the registry fee—I am still writing my thesis, he is picking up shift work—and I haven't bought anything new to wear. Instead, I pull from the back of my cupboard a lilac-gray day dress from the forties, which I bought on eBay years ago, with a wide high neck and dolman shoulders that come down to tight princess sleeves. The Turkish woman at the milk bar is bringing the waist in for me; I am collecting it tomorrow, a few hours before the ceremony.

She stashes away the fabric, and we talk, and I forget about my eyebrows, and I steal slices of Parmesan cheese from the block while she cooks dinner. The next morning I pick up my dress, and whatever has happened to it has brought the hem up above my knees, much too high for its lines, but it is too late to make changes; in my little navy spotted veil, and green pickle of a coat, and orange-red lipstick, I feel like one of Monet's watercolors, floating on the surface of my own nerves.

Helen meets me outside the treasury building with a bouquet of lilac roses she has brought as a surprise, taking all the right tones from the piece of fabric I gave her. They are my "something new." Inside, she reads a poem while Mike and I hold hands, as ordered by the celebrant, who also insists on "a little light classical music" tinkling through the stereo, though we are happy to just sign the papers and go get a coffee. An Indian bridal party has booked the room after this, and the grandmother of the bride keeps poking her head in to see if we are done yet. Amazingly, incredibly, we soon are.

When our marriage becomes public, Helen comes over with a small wrapped gift, and although it is from her whole family, I know that she has chosen it herself. It is a painting by Sean, and it is perfect—exactly the right thing.

The title is scrawled on the back: *Altered Night*, Sean Bailey. Despite our small collection, it is only with this painting that the strange and deep responsibilities of owning art come home to me. Up until this point I have been fairly blithe with the few paintings we have, not yet rearranging my mind-set about art from it being something that goes in public museums, *for everyone*, to something that has been entrusted to *me*.

It is beautiful and a little terrifying. The painting itself I love immediately. The figurative aspect is a mountain or geode on a pale, pale blue ground, and it carries a tension between the precision of its outlines, the half-obscured collage aspects receding from their overworking paint, and the vividly halted gestural qualities of the materiality of the painting's surface. More than anything, it is a painting that is perfectly still; that stillness I try to take, and keep inside me, as I look.

This stillness or, rather, a refusal of temporality, is the

thing I love most about painting. In any other art form—
dance, music, and in some visual art itself—you are moved
along in time as the art itself unfolds; even reading presupposes a dual movement along a line of text and forward
through time—it is constantly ongoing and exhausting.
But painting, no matter how full of "movement" it is, exists
in the blink of an eye or over the course of a century, in
and of itself exactly the same. Contexts change, moods
change, the knowledge that we bring to bear on it changes,
but the object itself is finite; movement is stilled; rework-
ing is impossible; it is done.

I find Sean's paintings so beautiful and so restful. In
the course of a move I hang this one on a hook that promptly
falls off the wall, and a tiny bit of its patina is chipped away,
revealing a minute speck of board. My first instinct is to
apologize to the work, and I do, and then I take it and hold
it in both hands and survey the damage, which is visible
only to me. Any responsibility I have felt toward this work
immediately triples. Now that I have hurt it, I have need
to love it even more.

This stillness and sense of peace I try to keep within me as
I lose my own ability to work. For a while, Helen and I
are traveling in tandem. Heavily pregnant, I sit on her floor
in the sharehouse and drink a small glass of red, just one,
the heater on, shoes off, and my feet encased in the feet of
my maternity tights. We are proofreading the second edition of her contemporary art journal, launched the previous

year—a brilliant, typically Helen endeavor that has replaced advertising with artists' pages, and rejects any relationships with the major private galleries.

My belly gets in the way of the print proofs; I have to wiggle around to see them. A few of us work in comfortable, companionable silence, occasionally asking questions about the spelling of surnames, or whether "Centre" should be spelled as "Center" in particular American contexts. I am happy to be engaged in this work, to give my time; a few years earlier, I had launched my own small journal with my friends Gillian and Caroline, an experimental fashion and design magazine that sailed right into the winds of the financial crisis and was shipwrecked there. Helen lent me a dress for the launch; there is nothing she hasn't given me.

She comes to visit Owen in the hospital, one of a few beloved visitors. As he grows, and I grow ill, she embarks on her PhD, juggling teaching and research with her paid work, and falling out of love, and falling in love again. She visits as much as she can, but our lives have gone along different pathways, and her life is very full; more and more we rely on text message exchanges, which I send while Owen is breastfeeding—the only time he does not try to grab the phone.

As I drop out and stop being able to write, or draw, or concentrate, Helen throws herself into volunteer endeavors and art fairs and publishing; she gets up early in the morning to write extra essays and articles, whereas I am up because there is a little Klaxon in my house keeping me awake. Sean's painting presides over a living room that is covered with unfolded laundry, half-drunk cups of tea, baby toys, more toys, so many things underfoot. I am living in a world that is half adult, half utterly infantile.

Occasionally, if I stop to think about it, I envy her for how much farther ahead of me she seems to be getting. I feel as though my life is in stasis; not the beautiful, still poetry and peace of Sean's painting, but *fucked*, in a way that hers is not fucked: for Helen, there is still mobility. She can throw a big dinner party and stay up late; she can go to the Sydney Biennale on a whim, or organize a symposium about its ethics when asked to.

I do not begrudge her these things. I have seen how hard she has been working, and I love her, and the more she forges ahead the more I am proud of her, proud to know her, not exactly living vicariously through her successes, but taking a pleasure in them that goes way beyond the pleasures of my own static life. Like Hustvedt's split subject, I seem to have severed myself, but instead of a "self-reflective distance," I am only achieving distance from the self *as is*, a turning away. What I see, reflected in Helen, is myself as I could be, not as I am. And I wonder if I will ever be fit to travel alongside her again.

In the druggy, icy morning, after Mike has gone to work, I pull Owen into bed with me and put on an episode of *Play School*. Bright, competent, cheery voices fill the room, and I burrow back into a half-sleep, one hand clutching Owen's foot to make sure he is still there.

On *Play School*, ordinary objects are transmuted, often into other ordinary objects. Transformation is low-key and recognizable. A shoe box becomes a car; Jemima dresses up as a monkey; art is posited as nonthreatening and achievable. There is no ecstasy in this, just safety. I long for the unexpected physical sensations of art; of walking into a gallery and standing transfixed, experiencing a suspension in temporality and even in space; a narrowing of the perimeters of the world until all that is left is the plane of air between my eyes and someone else's work. This is a space in which the body disappears, irritations disappear; the eyes are satiated, the self is awash in color or texture or form. In more craven terms, I am longing for escape.

As I lie in bed, half-sleeping, and Owen is enraptured by Luke and Leah or Justine and Jay, I am aware of an extremely rudimentary therapy taking place. My psychiatrist at the hospital has suggested that childbirth is a kind of second adolescence, a knock back to a time charged with hormones and uncertainty and new psychological growth. I feel knocked back further, all the way to infancy, about as psychologically fit as the child sitting next to me, though he is all of a piece; his horizons are limited, he doesn't know what he is missing.

Art therapy is a widely practiced approach, of course, though its applications vary. During a depressive episode, the limbic system is compromised, specifically the amygdala, the thalamus, and the hippocampus. In a study of women, the hippocampus of those who have experienced depression is shown to be nine to thirteen percent smaller than that of those who haven't.[2] The more depression experienced, the smaller the hippocampus. Visual stimulus can renew and strengthen neural pathways here; think of a photograph "retrieving" a memory; the plasticity of the brain is to its benefit in reforging connections.

In a study conducted in Israel, researchers found a statistically significant reduction in the symptoms of depression among mothers suffering from postpartum depression when psychotherapy was supplemented with art therapy. The study is framed in terms of a cost-benefit analysis; as in Australia, the Israeli mental health-care system is a shambles. I like the frankness with which their findings are summed up in the abstract:

> In a health care system with chronic budgetary
> constraints, the addition of some cardboard and
> plasticine to the "Health Basket," coupled with a
> few hours with a trained therapist, is probably a
> worthy alternative, considering the scope of the
> problem and its influence on the mother, the
> baby, and the family as a whole.[3]

The bits of publishing-world gossip that get back to me deplore the unexpected sales spike in coloring books for adults. My friend Mel disparages them as pandering to the "adult baby" market, and I can see her point: they are marketed with wholesale condescension, sprinkled with the buzzwords of *mindfulness* and *stress reduction*; they manage to reduce genuine mental health approaches down to the size of a box of Derwents. My mum firmly frowned upon coloring-in when I was a child; we were given sheets of butcher paper and markers, or on sunny days sent outside to chalk up the garden walls. But I can see the appeal of something prescriptive, to keep the hands occupied. At the very least, they probably do no harm.

Amrita Sher-Gil does not have any children of her own. Her entire body of work is created before she is as old as I am now; she dies at the age of twenty-eight, shockingly, shockingly young. There is some suspicion of her husband, Victor, having murdered her, but more likely it was a failed abortion, and attendant peritonitis, a fatal inflammation of the membranes of the abdomen. She slips into a coma a few days before her first major show, and never wakes up to see her work arranged, admired, institutionalized.

I think of her life, so compressed but so vivid in its scope, and wonder what she would have made if she had lived; whether she, too, would have been paralyzed by the advent of children. I wonder, if she did have an abortion, how much of her decision was inspired by the fear that she would have to give her life over, even briefly, to stasis, tedium, grime. I look at the lives of famous artists and count the number of children that they have, like Roland Barthes in "Novels and Children,"[4] but counting the children does not give me any clue to how these women are feeling.

When I begin to recover, when Owen is too large to be brought like a hibernating mouse in his sling to book launches and readings, but still far too small not to need me, I begin to come up against the difficulties of being an artist-mother. It is not just now that I am foundering, faltering in my mind and with no time to write, but that there is no room in my larger writing life for a baby or small child. There are no writers' residencies where babies are welcome; few conferences provide childcare on-site, and none of the hip coworking spaces that spring up in my neighborhood are child-friendly.

I am tangling with a new, unspoken etiquette: the sense that the polite thing to do is put my head down, stay home, attend to my child, and reappear after a few years, when my life more easily molds to the pattern of six p.m. book launches and countless hours of unpaid arts-organization overtime—just disappear, and come back as though nothing has changed me or changed the pace of my life. I am too tired to rock the boat, but it is difficult making work this way, and, above everything else, it is lonely.

To write, even if you can, is to take the risk that you will remain unread—that nobody's eyes or mind will animate your words, or breathe with them, unconsciously, in their own idiosyncratic way. I am scared that everything I make will remain dead marks on a page. I ache for the ability to take something material, move swiftly within its sphere, and to have it comprehended in an instant. I try to tell Helen some of this, and she disappears for a moment and comes back with a volume of Michael Fried.

"Let me read you the most perfect paragraph," she says:

This preoccupation [with duration] marks a profound difference between literalist work and modernist painting and sculpture. It is as though one's experience of the latter *has no* duration—not because one *in fact* experiences a picture by Noland or Olitski or a sculpture by David Smith or Caro in no time at all, but because *at every moment the work itself is wholly manifest* . . . It is this continuous and entire presentness, amounting, as it were, to the perceptual creation of itself, that one experiences as a kind of *instantaneousness*, as though if only one were infinitely more acute, a single infinitely brief instant would be long enough to see everything, to experience the work in all its depth and fullness, to be forever convinced by it.[5]

When I speak of Amrita, I know that she is dead. But to me, she exists continually in the present, alive in death, because this is the space that she has made: a continuous and entire presentness that contracts and expands like a heart.

If I am to visit Amrita in her studio in 1941, will I find her pacing, chewing the ends of her paintbrush, agonizing over a color that won't come good? Perhaps she has an embryo nestling in the soft tissue of her womb; perhaps she knows about it, perhaps there are twinges of pain that she thinks are a kidney infection, or maybe she puts her nausea down to the drenching Lahore heat.

Maybe she is laid still and stagnant, too, sometimes, from the heat or from sadness or from causes that I cannot glean. I know that to look in from the outside is not to see the all of how she lives, and I cannot count her happiness by the number of her paintings.

I know, too, that I should not fetishize the stillness that I find in her work, because of course the urge to work and work over the material surface of a painting must be as compelling as the urge to write and rewrite until something is perfect. For when we take our hands off, when we lift the brush, how are we to know that we have not finished forever?

Helen is turning thirty now, and soon I will be, too. It feels as though a minute ago I was standing on a piano stool at her twenty-first-birthday party, making a tipsy, impromptu speech. When we move house, she gives us a collage on permanent loan, a beautifully odd figure of a shaman that I have always admired. He goes with us everywhere—"For good luck," Helen says.

She is beginning to think about having a baby herself, and so once again we are traveling down parallel paths. We used to joke about our littlest siblings, Edward and Olivia, falling in love and having babies, and about our own children growing up as best friends like we did, but life doesn't unfold itself tidily like that. I can manage the small things: going to the launch of the latest issue of her magazine, *Discipline*, which is acclaimed now and thriving; texting her at ten in the morning with a photograph of a haircut I might like to get; cheering her on from afar as she gets gussied up to collect her PhD, her cheekbones and her father's identically wide in beaming, wonderful smiles.

I return to Hustvedt's essay, thinking about intersubjectivity. Beyond neurological development, she moves through philosophy and into an engagement with the intentionality of art, its physicality, but always comes back to the idea of the mirror:

> The reflective quality is there because we are
> witnessing what remains of another person's
> creative act, and through the artistic object we
> find ourselves embroiled in the drama of self and
> other. This back-and-forth dialectic between
> spectator and artwork occurs despite the fact that a
> painting, sculpture, or drawing is also just a thing,
> an object like any other in the material world . . .
> It is not a tool. We can't eat with it. Art is useless.[6]

To get a closer look at Sean's painting, I begin to weave a companion piece to it, gathering wools not in his vivid cobalt and dark violets—I don't have any on hand—but in my own preferred palette of pale slate blue, dark gold, sludge green. I try to break down into comprehensible little fractals the intense overlaying of colors in his painting—the place, not replicable at my very amateur skill level, where different layers of pigment merge or overlap. Then I go into the other room and begin to weave.

Owen loves watching me at the loom—"It's like a harp!" he says, running his fingers over the freshly laid warp—and sits at my side, occasionally trying to stick a piece of wool in to help me. I set him up with some oil pastels and paper, and he leans over in his chair, left hand grasping a pastel firmly, and frowning as he drags it across the page. His lines give me a pure, powerful happiness; it is wonderful to watch him work.

Side by side, we are sharing a singular concentration, caught together in much the same way I have found myself caught together with Helen or Mike when we are looking at a piece of art we both enjoy; as though the pleasure of looking is made stronger by the silent knowledge that somebody else is looking, too.

Hustvedt's essay speaks to the intense, uplifting transportation of finding yourself suddenly communing with a work of art, but the question broadens out, for me, I think; it is not just that I am in contact with the traces of someone else's hand, but that I am near the physical, present body of someone who catches my unspoken thoughts as they travel toward a piece of art. As much as I like Sean, it is not him I am thinking of when I stand and look at *Altered Night*; though I see the presence of his hand, he isn't the first person posited in the dialectic of self and other.

Rather, it is my other self, my lifelong friend that I think about. On days when I feel very far away, I rest my eyes for a minute on the painting's deep, soothing blues. And I am warmed, as I always am, by Helen's generosity and affection and perfect taste—which is only, at its core, knowing someone more deeply than words, so that you can give them something that you know they will cherish for life.

WEAVING

THE WEFT ENCOMPASSES the warp in soft little puffy half-circles—*under, over, under, over*—then doubles back: *over, under*. Somewhere at the edge of vision, my child is playing with a toy truck. My husband is reading, and I can see the flicker of pages as my needle passes through the tight warp threads. Stillness, stillness, *flicker*.

My hair is clubbed up on the top of my head, out of the way—it has grown long enough to get in the way again. A small ache runs up my back and settles in my shoulders. I try to bend from the waist, pull my shoulders down, and breathe softly, so as not to jar my rib cage, dredging as much of that softness as I can into my hands.

All of my body is now in my fingertips. The weft encompasses the warp, and hides it, gradually, in growing spans of cloth. Colors flit past each other and rest on the edges I have drawn, not straightforwardly, but in staircase configurations of interlocks and slits. The feeling of wool beneath my hands is almost unbearably sensual. It has taken me so long to get here.

I hadn't woven for maybe twenty years when I fell pregnant, and then it wasn't wool, but paper. I remember, vividly, threading bright strips of craft paper through a precut template, the kind of activity that kindergarten teachers prepared the night before, fifteen or twenty at a time.

Weaving with paper is a good metaphor for the bulk of my creative life, which itself is shot through with metaphor: the language of weaving is so much a part of the fabric of speech that it goes almost unnoticed. To spend my life writing is to spin a yarn; I weave two threads of a narrative together, untangle or unsnarl a linguistic problem, embroider a fact. The words *text* and *textile* come from a common source, the Latin *texere*, meaning to construct or weave, either a story or a cloth.

The metaphors of weaving don't stop at creation. Particularly, one can unravel, if one finds oneself at a loose end. Cloth that slips off the loom is liable to fray if it is not finished off neatly, and one can drop stitches, as in knitting, and find a fatal negative imprint in space that only grows the longer it is unattended. A person can be too highly strung, become warped.

. . .

When I first begin to lose my connection to words, I don't believe that anything serious is going on. Temporary aphasia is a fairly common symptom of pregnancy, part of the catchall "baby brain" that excuses clumsiness, forgetfulness, teariness.

Language is my bread and butter, but I am lucky: I am working at a magazine where the editor and I are so silently sympathetic that sometimes we can go entire days without real conversation. If I drop a word, it is usually only into his outstretched hand.

Patrick is gracious, but I catch him looking faintly quizzical at times and recall myself to myself in the middle of a sentence, one in which I've unconsciously substituted a poorer word for the right one, skipping over meaning for the closest possible sound.

"I did it again, didn't I?" I ask, and he has to say yes.

Unraveling is a painful process, one that rapidly outpaces my ability to repair the damage. When Owen is born, the vocabulary lost to the pregnancy doesn't suddenly flood back, as I had half expected, certainly hoped. Instead, the process of deterioration speeds up, leaving me exhausted by attempts to keep up with the train of my most basic thoughts.

Unraveling itself is a trick, with *raveling* its synonym and antonym. You can reconcile them by thinking of a loom;

the *unraveling* threads, becoming unwoven from the fabric, are *raveled*, tangled up.

I can't think of anything much in particular. I can keep up the flow of social conversation, a beat behind the others who come to coo at the baby, but it exhausts me, leaves me cranky and tired. I am tired physically, tired emotionally, sick of not being able to find the right word at the right time, and terrified that I will never be able to find it again.

Language is where I have lived for so long, I am lost without it. When I read, the words make no impression on my brain, vanishing before I finish a paragraph, so that I have to read it again and again to glean its meaning. It is like my life before glasses; language becoming, with strain, simply a gray blur across the page.

It is truly fucking horrific, and the irony is that I have no words left to describe it.

The bookshelves are stuffed with books I bought as a student, which I no longer flip through, no longer understand. A lot of them center on psychoanalytic criticism, my chosen branch of theory; I can remember thoughts darting through these like a kingfisher across the surface of a lake, picking up bits of knowledge as easily and intuitively as a bird hunts fish.

I loved the French theorists in particular, though they weren't untroubled, especially Jacques Lacan. I have never felt that Freud's reduction of the world into sex is persuasive, but I love the way in which Lacan reconfigures existence into something made up predominantly of language. This is how I have always seen the world: as being made up of, created by, words. In Lacan's structure, the world is tripartite, consisting of three realms he calls the Imaginary, the Symbolic, and the Real, and these three are irretrievably locked together in a Gordian knot.

The Real, contra its name, is a fantasy world, where the dark and dangerous, too terrifying for language, go to play. The Imaginary is a preliterate soup of desire and the fulfilment of desire, a kind of infant's paradise of lust, longing, piquancy, and joy. It is a space we leave behind in order to enter the Symbolic, the world of language and schemes, where words delineate a common understanding and are exchanged freely in a shared, communal conception of existence. That is the trade-off—to narrow the world to language, in order to share it with others.

Now that language is eluding me, I am shunted between states, no longer feeling in common with any aspect of the world. My infant child lives wordlessly, and I begin to follow him in wordlessness. There is no consolation there, only loss; you can never go home again, to the Imaginary world, and without the schema of language I am amorphous, adrift.

I do manage to put this into words one day, imperfectly, in a forty-five-minute window of blessed lucidity. The online editor of my old lit mag, *Going Down Swinging*, has asked me for some work, and somehow, during Owen's nap, I make it, word after word after word, only eight hundred or so, but for the time while I am making it, an exalted time; I am afraid to twitch, to leave the desk. Something is flowing through me that is filling me with light.

Owen wakes, and the spell is broken. A few weeks later the piece is published, and swiftly I receive an invitation to perform at a spoken word night across the river. I struggle to read the email through a dampening, wordless fog, and wonder what the convener of that night has read and what he has understood.

For my birthday, Mike hands me a small camera.

"Perhaps this will help you feel creative again," he says, giving me a kiss.

For months I have been ossified, unable to write, unable to think beyond the immediate needs of the house and the baby and my husband and my job, a new job, mostly administrative but still in the arts.

I think back to the drawing class I took while I was pregnant, determined to eke out some time for myself between work and home, a small pause in the day.

The first night I draw a pumpkin, and all of my buried knowledge floods back into my hands. I take the drawing home and tack it to the cupboard door. It will be the best thing I draw during that class; my belief in my facility ebbs as I grow bigger, and clumsier, and soon unable to stand at an easel for a prolonged period of time.

The baby whacks my kidneys with impatience when I sit at the table at night, trying in vain to capture the spontaneity and basic firmness of those first clear lines. *Why bother*, the kicks seemed to say, *why bother to make anything but me.*

Now, with the camera in my hands, I try to see the world afresh. I set myself a deadline—a photo every Friday—and start a blog, *Empty Eye*, taking the name from *The Backward Shadow*: "I felt the empty eye of advance grief opening up inside me like a lens."[1]

All I can see, when opening myself up to glimpse the world, is my own inadequacy. From my hands come lines that are stilted; from the lens, images that are clichéd, poorly framed, unbalanced in composition and color and tone. Drawing and photography, though I try to force myself to think of them as mechanical acts, are intimate, subjective, and my subjectivity is shattered into tiny, tiny pieces.

I see a psychologist, Anita, under the auspices of a low-cost program for women in my new suburb. We have moved from my beloved Footscray now, relying more and more on my mother to help raise our child. When I am with him, I am in danger of being swallowed whole.

Anita is pregnant herself, her comfortable jersey dresses stretching out over a stomach that becomes larger with every visit. She is a cellist, and understands the problem, but in a way that leaves me feeling as though we are speaking different languages.

"I can't write," I tell her, trying to convey how deeply

the problem goes. My face is as still as a mask. "I feel as though I am corroding."

"What's this 'corroding'?" she responds. "Why do you say that? It is still there, you know, it is just under a layer of dust. You need to wipe the dust off to see it clearly. Do you expect to be wonderful right when you are coming back to it? No! You need to practice!"

I wonder briefly if she is right, if what I am experiencing is just writer's block, a frustration with my inability to get it right straight off the bat, what another therapist will call "a schema of unrelenting high standards." But I know she is wrong, because of the feeling of my core being eaten by rust.

As a musician she has a safeguard—a physical barrier between her subjective self and her interior expressions of music, and her outward expression of the same. But thought is language is writing is words; apart from the mechanism of the mouth, or maybe fingers, it pours out directly without mediation, with no protective translation of inner self into music, image, cloth.

If only I could translate this lack, this corrosive inability to think and be, into *something*, I think—perhaps I might be okay.

One of my favorite stories as a child was the story of Theseus and the Minotaur, the man facing off against the beast. I liked its secret hero, Ariadne, who gives Theseus a spool of thread and tells him to unravel it as he enters the

Labyrinth, so that he can follow it safely outside again. Ariadne almost certainly knows how to weave, as does poor Arachne, turned into a spider for her pride.

My friend Leah lends me Taschen's *Book of Symbols*, where I meet Arachne again. Leah is a photographer who is also not working, and we meet in the Botanical Gardens for long strolls in the twilight before I dash off to pick up Owen from childcare. We talk about what it is to be outcast from our work, how strange and inarticulable the world seems without the ability to transform it, or reveal it, through our lost sources of metamorphosis and change.

From time to time Leah inspects a succulent, paying particular attention to where new growth is budding, or old scars healing over with sap. In her tiny apartment in the heart of the city she is growing a garden, regenerating hardy plants from torn-off leaves she's found in green patches all over town. Her cats have learned to leave these scraps alone. They are named Shrigley and Arbus, and curl together in the midday sun.

"What botany does for one woman, weaving does for another," Leah writes, posting an image of my first completed weaving hanging over her propagation table. I have made it for her with the Mornington Peninsula, where she grew up, in mind, trying to capture its silvery mix of ghost gums and agapanthus, scrubby ground cover and sea.

It hangs over the tables for a full hour before one of the cats discovers it. After that it is moved to a higher spot, away from her small jars of cuttings.

. . .

I see a new therapist, Kristy, months later when the problem hasn't resolved itself. She's a practitioner at the clinic my new psychiatrist runs. She is warm and calm and blond and groomed, somebody I like as a woman as well as a psychologist. She is easy to talk to. Because I can't help myself, I have a go at the painting on her wall, a branch of blossom done in pale colors spacked on by a palette knife. I think it is terrible; Kristy tells me, again calmly, that she enjoys looking at it. I admire her for the way she puts me in my place without making me feel small.

"What would you do," she asks me, "if you could no longer write?"

I take a minute to digest the question. I find that I literally cannot conceptualize the future she is talking about, one in which my work and, sometimes I think my vocation, is firmly in the past.

"Couldn't write, or couldn't do anything creative?" I hedge.

"Let's say anything creative."

I think of a life without writing, photography, doodling little scribbles with Owen; without making up stories for him or funny little songs, without singing with Mike of an evening while he plays the guitar, without a joy in cooking or arranging spring flowers in a vase or painting a wall pale celery green.

"I don't think," I say, "that I *could* live."

"Well," says Kristy, leaning forward, "we had better work on that."

The physical weaving comes almost by accident. The pockets of lucidity grow longer, and the editor of a newspaper's lifestyle supplement gets in touch, having read something I've written long ago for an indie magazine. I pitch her a story about craft weaving, having sat up night after breast-feeding night staring at my phone, watching a glut of tapestries fill my Instagram feed and wondering at their provenance and sudden ubiquity.

I enroll in a course a stylist is hosting in a warehouse space in Prahran. Among thirty or so women, I sit quietly and anonymously, ears out for any telling snippets of conversation that could be threaded into an article. In writing, you call this "color"; in the vast room color abounds, in the piles and piles of wool heaped around large tables, the bright clothes of the instructors, the glittery special yarns that two older women refer to as "bling." I like them instinctively. One winds the bling yarn around her iPhone again and again, just the right length to cut for rya knots in a fringe.

I try to find a deeper connection here, to the second-wave feminist craft movements of the 1970s, and to spiritual, mythical, and archetypical ideas of women's craft. The conversation, though, stays on the surface, perhaps because my brain is rusty, perhaps because these particular works are being made in emulation of something, a trend in interiors that bubbles up and then dies down. The physical part of it is easy. It's a skill even I can learn.

After I file the article, I begin to find an underground. It reassures me that there are women—mostly women—who have trained, worked, held to this craft for years, and are steadily seeing out its popularity by turning their backs on a trend and setting fiber to its course. One of them, a tapestry weaver in Geelong, sends me a link to a bloody Norse epic in which women pull the guts out of the enemy and construct a massive loom, weighting it down with the heads of dead men. It is thrillingly visceral, and seems to turn my blood.

The warp encompasses the weft, but weaving is an interpenetration, a locking together of threads. Rachel, the weaver from Geelong, works sideways, her deft fingers possessing a confident foreknowledge of the final work, weft turning to warp and warp to weft. The final pieces are beautiful, and I yearn to reach through the screen of my phone and touch them.

Leah and I meet up again, planning a trip to the museum. I often sneak an hour in the National Gallery of Victoria, wallowing in art, but since having a small inquisitive boy I have been reminded about natural history. I would be happy lounging on Leah's floor, playing with watercolors and snuggling her cats, but she needs to get out of the house, and the museum, on a concession card, is free.

We spend about half an hour in the indoor rain forest,

breathing in the richly oxygenated air and wending our way up the path, looking at spiders and frogs and reading about their various species, the largest and smallest ferns, and the shoots now regenerating from Black Saturday's devastating flames. The museum is big, so we decide to pick one exhibition and spend a while loitering in it.

I vote for the rocks, a visit to walls and walls of mineral formations: the sparkling quartzes, shales, and malachites; the meteor glass formed when stellar debris hit desert sand. Leah gravitates to minerals in shades of pale pink and golds; I like the sludgy mud greens and acidic yellows, and the colors in between—chartreuse and mustard—of minerals with high sulfur content.

Afterward, Leah takes me to a wool shop that has opened in an arcade near her flat, and laughs when we realize that I am drawn here, too, to green, she to pink. Her choices aren't precious or babyish, but the colors of spun sugar or sun hitting beach salt in the very late afternoon. I buy a hank of rock-gray roving, wool that has been carded but not yet spun, and a thick ball of murky green wool shot through with bronze, egged on by Leah, who is enjoying vicariously the act of impulse buying.

Together we wander the shop and run our hands, lightly, over irresistible textures. I am surprised to be able to tell her from the touch whether a ball of wool is alpaca or merino, whether it is pure or blended with silk, and explain the process by which felt is made. There are knowledges my hands have been internalizing, and it's gratifying to share them with someone who lives so keenly in her senses.

There is such joy in the physicality of this, the slow materialization of an object under my fingers. I revel in its tactility, the stash of wool that I am accumulating in an old picnic basket kept high up, where Owen can't reach.

I become a magpie, swooping down on each ball of wool I come across to determine its suitability in a future weaving. Every op-shop I visit has a stash of eight-ply somewhere: usually a few odds and ends of bright synthetics, but sometimes the true pure wool of whites, sands, and creams.

At night, I sit and wrestle with my basic notched frame, trying to prop it up on something to spare my back. Mike sits with me, boxboard and pens and ink arranged around him, gently making fun of me as he draws.

As I struggle to keep tension, his pen swoops across the page, creating images that are unmistakably his. Mike's drawing comes out of nowhere seemingly, blossoming up after a few years together. One day he buys a sketchbook and fills it with the figures of tourists, sketching in loose but strong lines that have an immediate coherence.

It seemed to me a minor miracle that one could start, and continue, with a clear and steady voice; to not fumble around searching for it, but feel it inborn in you.

He shows me a sketch of our conversation:

"I think you're getting really good."

"Eh, I think I have a way to go."

"But the weavings you did before are great!"

"But you can't see what's inside my brain!"

What I make in wool rarely reflects what exists in my mind's eye, but somehow this doesn't upset me. There is a calmness, a sureness to the motion of wool under warp that creates almost a trance state; in many weaving cultures, practitioners have believed that the soul can become trapped in the cloth, so hypnotic is the physical motion. The safeguard against this is to leave a small flaw in, to break the pattern of perfection. Flaws put in by mistake are immediate and apparent, easily remediable. Another miracle, to be able to see and fix quickly the things that need fixing.

Mike packs away his pens and paper.

"I ran out of loom puns."

"What about the ill-loom-inati?"

He begins to sketch again.

Textile and *text*; they are more intimately linked than even I know. I trade weaving with writing, turning to one to soothe the defects of the other when I need a consolation—*subject* to *object*, *ephemeral* to *material*.

Like *raveling* and *unraveling*, they are antonyms and also synonyms. I come across a book by Kathryn Sullivan Kruger, now so pricey in the printed volume that I read it in PDF though I long to hold it in my hands, called *Weaving the Word: Metaphorics of Weaving and Female Textual Production*. It is just what I need, and I marvel at its existence.

Kruger confirms my hunch about the metaphors permeating language, the physical act of weaving so unfamiliar to most of us now that the metaphors have come unmoored. She writes of the common source of language and weaving in myth: of the African Dogon, whose ancestor, Nummo, wove the very first word of language against the teeth of his mouth, a giant loom; of the Navajo Spider Woman, who "conceives all beings, stories, and every aspect of the natural world in her mind and on her web"; of Isis, Ixchel, Tlazolteotle, Mokusa, female goddesses who support the work of weavers and often storytellers.

What unmoors me, though, is her generosity, her feminism. She writes:

> I propose that when we talk about literature
> and its history, we should also include in our
> discussion the ancient production of texts in the
> form of textiles (even if these texts via textiles
> survive only in the form of stories) . . . Writing
> was invented around fifty-five hundred years
> ago, and has only become a widespread practice
> in the last four hundred years or so. Before
> written texts could record and preserve the
> stories of a culture, cloth was one of the primary
> modes for transmitting these social messages.
>
> Moreover, when reestablishing the connection
> between the written text and the textile, we
> must also concede that there exists a significant
> relationship between women, who wove textiles,

and textual production. By recuperating a textile
history and including it in our awareness of
literary history, we will recover a large community
of female authorship.[2]

This staggers me, moves me almost to tears. For so long I
have felt cast out of my own authorship, void of voice. To
think simply that my fingers are moving in a long tradition of signification, that marks in wool are the natural pre-
cursors to marks on a page, shifts the world sideways for
me into sense.

Later, in her work, Kruger draws on Lacan's and Kristeva's theories pertaining to abjection of the mother body,
and my knowledge of Lacan and the Symbolic and the Real
are right there in my mind, clean and polished and accessible. It is incalculable richness to swim in the tides of critical theory, which I thought had ebbed far out, forever.

There is another passage my mind keeps coming back to,
when I put my fingers to the loom, that is simpler, perhaps
the crux of it. In Rumer Godden's memoir, she writes of a
book she was working on years after she lost her first child,
a stillborn boy:

"It occurs to me," says the hero of the book,
"that we were put into this world as a part of its
making, as a stitch or a thread is put into the
weaving of a cloth or tapestry. When we die

we leave a little hole and it is our duty, before we
die, to see that the hole is filled and so strengthen
the weave."

I had written that when Jane was on the way
and I wonder if it was why I longed so much for
another child.[3]

I am lucky, truly lucky, to have one beautiful, funny,
inquisitive child, but his infancy is shot with loss; there are
holes that may never be filled. With my loss of language
came an attendant loss of memory, and, trying to reach
my mind back, there are stretches of time that are simply
inaccessible.

I do not even realize, sometimes, that my memory is
gone. The mind plays tricks, picking up loose edges and
tying them up so neatly they give the appearance of continuity. That sense of continuity is probably needed, and saving, but occasionally Mike will say something that frays the
protective congruence—*I'm craving that sourdough we used to
buy*—and suddenly vistas open up: I do remember that
bread! The sourdough bread that each week I walked a ki-
lometer and a half each way to buy, trekking the distance
between Footscray and Seddon with Owen in the pusher,
and then doubling back when I realized, every time, that
he had taken off his left shoe and thrown it out the side.

I wonder if some of this compulsion toward materiality
comes from the fact of these lacunae; that no matter how I
try to compensate, there will always have been a time in
his life when I was not *there*, not loving or present. And

there is nothing that I can do with the guilt I carry for that. It is simply, always, there, a little hole in the weave.

I try hard not to hover, to continue on my own path, not to smother him but keep healing, so that the force of my love is not too little or too much. At my place at the table, warping up my loom, I try to fasten into it the knowledge of making that resides in my fingers, and the urge to create that somehow connects me to my child. The wool in my hands is soft against skin that has been toughening, and smells very faintly of lanolin.

The movement of my electric-blue plastic tapestry needle is steady and practiced. Again, I slow my breathing, try to focus on the task at hand. Bit by bit the tapestry grows, and I make sure to leave in at least a single imperfection, so that my soul can escape the cloth and flow back to my body once more.

VIRGINIA'S SCARF

IN THE MONTHS after Virginia died, I often thought I saw her on the street. Walking Owen to day care, we would pass a woman in her sixties or seventies, and I would catch a glimpse of nautical stripes, or large gold earrings, or a dark bob streaked with gray, and for a second Virginia's face would superimpose itself on the face of a perfect stranger. After death, memory begins to ossify, fixing a person in time and space, but Virginia, in my mind, had long been static; unbending and unyielding, not much given to change. That is how I always thought of her—impervious— and maybe that was why she could appear so strikingly on the faces of other women.

I see her sometimes in photos, of my mother and myself, in a wry, grim set of the mouth that tells the photographer to *get on with it*. In candid shots our long necks are graceful and our slim shoulders roll forward, our mouths gentle and relaxed. We are most often watching others, carrying trays, holding babies: a quiet audience and domestic machinery, and perhaps this is why our faces in portraits are so embarrassed and defiant. Or maybe it is more simple: nobody ever taught us how to gracefully become the center of attention. The photographs in Virginia's house, long gone now, grouped us all as children, our names beneath our faces in dark blue ink.

If I close my eyes and enter the house, I can visit it lucidly, the details never changing except for seasonally, as approved. The carpets are light, and the tiles are cool underfoot, a kind of beige slate that is polished, not dusty. In the kitchen, a wooden birdcage houses a wooden bird; the green velvet lounge suite is arranged around a hearth, a stack of logs set neatly in the grate, waiting to be lit. Walking to the back of the house, I can look out onto the garden, fringed in mammoth daisies, where a green shed houses my grandfather's model trains.

To the right, off the kitchen corridor, a long room splits in two, with children's drawings and wooden toys lining the sitting room to the left. The right side holds the Princess Bed, guest bedroom for us grandchildren, "princess" because of the long canopy that drapes and enfolds us in our sleep. There are snores coming from this room, not from sleeping children but from the old hound, Geordie, who wheezes loudly as he breathes. A tumor was excised from his throat and left its mark on his vocal cords, so that in his waking doggy life, he could never again hunt rats.

If I people the house, I see Virginia again, buttering white bread in the kitchen for sandwiches and passing plates over the counter for us children to arrange on the dining table. In this ghost house where everything exists at once, I add my grandfather, really stepgrandfather, Jim, bringing back the slight stoop of his shoulders, the nicotine-yellow cast of his white curly hair. Playing time forward and backward he has either nine or eight and a half fingers. His pinkie he lost to Dupuytren's contracture; the half was grated off with a block of cheese, he tells me, or run over on his tiny, delicate train tracks.

We arrange ourselves around the table, sitting on green-and-white-striped cushions that are tied to the dark chair seats with bows. It is Boxing Day, and Jim's sons and grandchildren crowd around the barbecue, burning sausages. The sausages split apart like Jim's finger, the skins giving way to soft raw flesh. One year Jim will succumb to lung cancer, and after that Virginia will sell the house, and someone else will move in and redecorate. Virginia's new house is functional, with no inscribed history. It is there that things finally begin to change.

There have been tests over the past few years, for thyroid problems and cholesterol. Virginia's weight has ballooned, but that might simply be from getting older; the waist of

her wedding dress is tiny, and her three daughters, as teen-
agers, were racehorse lean. At Christmas she goes in for
blood tests, and the results come back on New Year's Eve;
my mother telephones me and her voice is shaky.

"Hi, darling," she says on the phone. "I just wanted to
call and let you know that Grannie's test results came back
and it's not good news. She has lymphoma."

"Don't worry about tonight, then," I respond, or perhaps my first voiced thought is, "Shit, shit, shit." Mum has
offered to babysit Owen so that Mike and I can go to Leah's
party, but there are always parties. "Are you sure?"

"Bring him over," she says. "I want to see my baby,
and it will be good for you to get out of the house."

It *will* be good for me to get out. To go to a party requires showering, real clothes, puncturing the apathy that
has grounded me in the house. I know that Mum is anxious to see me better, that her heart is punched with worry
for how flat and tired I have been, how joyless. She has saved
me again and again, driving over from the other side of
town with flowers, fresh food, abundant love.

Like the ghost of the holiday, a memory floats up: myself at thirteen or fourteen years old, sobbing on the Princess Bed with great racking breaths. My parents are heading
to a party in Red Hill; they have dropped us three girls off
to spend the night with Virginia and Jim and their sons,
a tradition; Jim is Scottish and always celebrates Hogmanay,
the Scottish New Year. At midnight one of the sons will
knock at the door and be first-foot-in; there will be whis-
key, haggis, tattie scones, and phone calls to Scotland. All

I know is that I am breaking through my skin with misery, wretched at being dumped like a child at my grandparents' when what I want is to spend the night at home, by myself.

I try to be quiet and separate and plead a headache, so as not to spoil it for everyone. Sometimes when I feel this violent unhappiness, I can lie down until it passes. It is depression, of course, which has hung over me like a shadow since my early childhood, but right now it is called moodiness, adolescence; I can't explain how these deep slips into alienation and despair differ from *being moody*, and I don't know, in fact, if they do. I try to keep myself apart, but my mother comes in and tries to jolly me out of it, sympathetic, which is fuel on the fire, of course.

"You know," she says, "once, a boy I knew asked me if I'd like to go to a party with him on New Year's Eve. I spent the entire night by myself at home, waiting for the phone to ring."

"Is that supposed to *console me*?" I demand, seething.

The more she tries to empathize, the angrier I become. Virginia hovers outside the door, waiting to make everything calm again, bring me a cup of Horlicks, offer brisk comforting phrases; I don't stop to think about her generosity in keeping us, only how much I don't want to be there, how much I loathe the unchanging closeness of her home. Mostly, I am terrified of being told to *pull my socks up*, Virginia's cure for any fit of what could be construed as self-indulgence—a short moment of sympathy, then a pragmatic, onward-Christian-soldiers solution.

I know, in this fit of volcanic grief over nothing, that I cannot pull my socks up; I cannot behave well, move forward, square my shoulders, keep a stiff upper lip. Though she has never directly said so, I feel as though my sensitivity is a faint embarrassment to Virginia: my dreaminess, my hunger to be counted as an adult, my blistering humiliations over seemingly nothing at all.

The mornings of lazing in front of the hearth at Virginia's house have dropped away; I forget about the little stash of children's books, the photos of us children, the afternoon she spent sewing a dozen different buttons, carefully chosen from a biscuit tin, onto the back pocket of my jeans. What I feel now are the scalding marks of her judgment, which never expresses itself as nastiness but rather impresses, through the force of her entire person, that there is a way that things are done, and that to press against the boundaries of that way is *getting above yourself* or *asking for trouble.*

I have become difficult, a difficult age, and our relationship has become difficult, too, mostly because I don't know how it is that I can love someone who I think disapproves of me, who makes me feel so constrained. Thinking about it ties me in knots, so I give myself over to sobs that leave me exhausted, emptied out, alone on the bed until I have no choice but to drag myself up and splash water on my eyes, trying to remember the words to "Auld Lang Syne."

Now, on the hot streets of Footscray, I squash the memory down. I will deliver Owen to my mother and give her a tight squeeze, eat dinner with her, and then catch the train with Mike into the city, pushing past revelers on the street to get to Leah's apartment. High up above Collins Street, I put everything deliberately out of mind and set about getting drunk, dancing with people I adore and making friends of people I don't know, working hard to sail through the evening on a note of elation and release.

I haven't seen Virginia much at all since having the baby. Part of it is geographic: I don't drive, and her house down on the peninsula is a public-transport nightmare. Friends of mine who grew up on the coast learned to drive early, bashing around the back roads lined with blue and white agapanthus. Getting to her house has always required a drive; it is too far to simply drop by.

Partly it is that I do not want her to see how little, how frighteningly little, I am coping. Terrified that she will *say something*, I don't give her the chance to show me any kindness or love.

Years beforehand, on the morning of Jim's funeral, my sister Olivia collapses in the hallway and is rushed to the hospital with what will turn out to be viral meningitis. The virus is traveling up her spine; my father drops Claire and me off at the church before he himself rushes to the emergency ward.

My mother isn't there, so Virginia takes my hand as we walk between the pews.

"Now, you just sit here next to me," she says. "I know that I can trust *you* not to go to pieces."

Claire sobs in the pew next to me as the priest goes through the service. I feel out of place in the Church of England, a sore thumb, and I try to find a semblance of grace in the modern stained glass. My throat is sore with pity as Jim's sons read the eulogy. The prayers are standard; when the priest begins to intone Corinthians 13, the New International Version, my mind follows it without conscious thought. It is our school hymn, in the older language, which I like much better than the new:

> Tho I speak with the tongues of men and of
> angels, and have not love, I am become as a
> sounding brass or a tinkling cymbal; and tho I
> have the gift of prophecy and understand all
> mysteries and all knowledge; and tho I have faith
> so that I can remove mountains, and have not
> love, I am nothing . . .

Virginia holds my hand firmly throughout the service. My aunt passes me tissues to pass to Claire; I have forgotten to bring them, and my mother's sleeve is very far away. I try not to think of Olivia in the emergency ward. It is amazing how small the box containing Jim seems.

I try to remember when Grannie became Virginia in my mind. My mother and her sisters, at Virginia's insistence, still refer to her as "Mummy." The name belongs to a time when women put a Sunday roast in the oven before church, and an apple cake in once the roast was out, for pudding. My grandfather Bob was a stock and station agent, who moved around the country with each promotion; I think now of Virginia alone in a house with three daughters, packing and cleaning for six weeks at a time while Bob went ahead to scout a new home.

Is she lonely? Or do the ladies she knows from church drop by to smoke in the kitchen with her? She will regret saying goodbye to the neighbors, this I know; everywhere she lives, mostly country towns, she makes an effort to get to know the neighbors. She will have to find a new hairdresser, a new butcher, a new school for her children, and sign herself onto new committees she does not, in fact, enjoy. There will be a new garden to tend, and a new rental oven with its own vagaries to master.

And all this time her daughters are growing, and my mother is growing reedy and slim, and sewing herself the only maxi skirt in town. She listens to Leonard Cohen and renames herself Suzanne; Susan, Sue, little Susie Q. She wears Virginia's wedding petticoat with desert boots, and smokes, and sunbathes topless at the quarry, planning for the day when she will go to college—the first in her family—and make a life for herself in Melbourne, in small terrace houses with parsley out the back.

I think of my mother as she was then, and marvel that she possessed the grace to grow away from Grannie's strictures; not defiant in any way but simply, organically, increasing the scope of her world. Instead of feeling squashed, made small by conservatism, she grew and grew, studying developmental psychology, sticking a vase of daisies next to the gearbox of her VW, and never once bringing home an Australian boyfriend.

Virginia's new house is built along the same lines as the old, with smaller and less characteristic proportions. One wing, slightly sunken, houses the lounge room, kitchen, and Virginia's bedroom and en suite. This is where she will spend most of her time, toward the end.

When the first prognosis is made, and my mother meets the oncologist, she turns to a friend for a second opinion. This friend is a professor of oncology; he looks at the scans and, kindly and without reservation, suggests palliative care. Virginia's oncologist is optimistic; he believes in chemotherapy. It is not up to us to suggest that Virginia should not fiercely, stubbornly cling to life, but the cancer is advanced, and there will not be much pleasure in the treatment. Since Jim died, she's become president of the Senior Citizens, organizing subsidized bus trips into Melbourne and getting a senior's discount on plants at the local nursery. When the chemo starts, her bustling will be stilled.

I know it is her choice, but I can't stifle a pang of irritation that she is so willing to defer to the oncologist, who seems to have his mind elsewhere, and who is only one busy, distracted man. Virginia's respect for authority and love of order means that doctors possess a capital *D* in her mind; he is Doctor, from a time when nurses and orderlies dropped the article: "Doctor will see you now." It is bright, it is impersonal, and it seems to have nothing to do with her swelling and aching flesh, her skin that has become papery-dry and irritated, her vanishing hair.

Another friend of my mother's—she is rich in friends—presses the keys of a beach house upon her. A twenty-minute drive from Virginia, my mother can be there now to soothe her hands with lotions, help ease her into bed, take her to appointments. The Princess Bed, stripped of its gauze, is in a small spare room with a new mattress, to prop up my mother and her youngest sister, who trade off nights in the house. Two puppyish beagles have taken Geordie's place, but now they go to lodge with my aunt, too much underfoot.

My mother and I drive down from Melbourne, where she has spent a few days catching her breath. Owen, in the backseat, burbles and yells, playing with a set of plastic rings. The new house is down behind another house, on a lot that has been subdivided horizontally, and it reveals itself slowly as we make our way down the drive. Mum pokes her head in as I wrangle Owen out of the car seat, snuggling him for a second to take in his fresh, clean scent.

Virginia is getting out of bed. I pop in to kiss her on the cheek.

"Oh, there you are," she says. "Why don't you put the kettle on and I'll be with you in a tick."

On the bedside table is a pamphlet about diffuse large

B-cell lymphoma, angled toward visitors and in shades of cloying pink. She nods toward it.

"Since becoming ill I've been telling everyone as much as I possibly can about this insidious disease."

I swallow a hiccup of laughter that is threatening to become hysterical, and put the kettle on. Only Virginia, I think, would speak of her own cancer like the host of a morning TV show, appointing herself community educator from the confines of her bed.

Owen is giggling in my mother's arms; she puts him down on the floor and he promptly tries to get up again, sticking his little bottom in the air and making his body into a bridge. Virginia rings a small set of bells, which makes him smile again and again, and imitates a kookaburra: *"Kook-kook-kook-kook-ca-ca-ca-ca-ca!"* Owen giggles, and she trills again, and I try to remember when I have ever seen her look so soft, so quiet, so at ease.

After tea and sandwiches, Virginia lies down on the bed again, and Owen plops down next to her. At eight months he is wriggly and squirming, but stays close in the circle of her arms, engrossed in a pair of sunglasses. I take a few photos of the three of them together, Susie and Virginia gazing at Owen adoringly as he chews and drools on the glasses and his toes, basking in the newness of him, the little bald patch on the back of his head, his weensy toenails, perfect mouth. I send a picture to my sister Claire, and she bursts into tears. She hadn't realized that Virginia has already shaved her head.

. . .

Virginia has decided that she will live until Owen's first birthday.

"I was planning on living until I was eighty-five," she says ruefully. She is seventy-eight now.

As she deteriorates, the bald skull is swathed in a series of soft turbans, small white cotton-silk blends that don't chafe the skin. Virginia's arms ache too much to tie up any scarves, but my aunt brings over some cotton-knit infinity scarves and loops them around her head. Denuded of her hair, the fineness of her cheekbones is brought out, and the firm shape of her jaw, which is hung with crepey skin. She looks bruised beneath the eyes, but her skin tone is even, almost glowing; chemotherapy buffs out the age spots and freckles that accumulate from a lifetime in the sun, slathered in tanning oil, and cigarettes smoked before cigarettes were bad for you.

My mother comes back from a visit close to tears. Virginia's mouth is lined with ulcers that have filled up with pus, and she has stoically endured them instead of letting anyone know. "Oh," says Virginia, "I didn't want to bother the hospital," or more likely, "I didn't want to be a nuisance." Mum's grief and sorrow are shot with exasperation, just below the surface, where I can see it seeping into the muscles of her neck. Soon she is sleeping at Virginia's house almost all the time, a change of clothes in the trunk of her car, and a bottle of Valium for emergencies.

. . .

As Virginia sinks, so does my mother, sometimes coming home from Virginia's via my house for a cup of tea and a hold of my child. It is out of her way, but she needs life, fresh new cooing life, and to do the things for me that she knows will make my life easier: to freshen the water in my flowers, sweep the kitchen floor, surreptitiously gather the toys from the bathtub and place them neatly on the rim. There are things here that she can straighten and tidy and put right; Virginia is too inherently a housekeeper, even ill, to need much done for her.

The beach house becomes my mother's refuge. We spend hours lying on the floor with Owen, listening to the whistle of the wind through the trees, watching rabbits dart across the lawn, and eating apples straight from the small orchard. Here, we pretend that we are on holiday, a little respite before the end, which despite Virginia's plans we both know is coming. There are conversations now about hospice care. The chemotherapy has been halted, palliative care finally instituted, enough for Virginia to regain her appetite, minutely; she and Owen subsist on purees and smooth dry biscuits, glasses of milk, finely sliced pieces of fruit.

Mum and I drive back from the beach, staying a night at Virginia's on our way home. I have a scarf knotted around my head like a turban to keep my hair out of my face, which Virginia likes. Her new walk-in robe is filled with large scarves, which she wears over her shoulders, dangling loose or held with a brooch. Now she is in a nightie and dressing gown, with leopard-print slippers that barely contain her swollen feet.

Soon it is evening, and Mum and I have forgone dinner, eating chocolate mousse out of plastic tubs with Virginia in front of the TV. Owen hangs off my breast, half asleep before he has had a chance to properly feed, and I tickle the bottom of his feet to wake him up again. He latches, and I close my eyes until I feel him drift off properly, then gather him up into the portable cot that Mum has set up in the study. "Four generations under the one roof," Virginia says.

Over the past few months, Mum and Virginia have been watching lifestyle television, *Selling Houses* and *Grand Designs*—any show that involves a full interior makeover in forty-five minutes. They know the names of the hosts, and nod sagely along to their advice. Occasionally one of us interjects. "Oh, I wouldn't have painted the front door in that color," says Virginia, looking at a fresh coat of scarlet designed to give a building "kerb appeal." "You can see that it will chip right off." Or: "I don't know if I would bother doing *that* to the banister."

We play a game, deciding which of the three houses being done up we would most like to live in, and the night falls silently outside, the screen flickering its reflected light in the windows, until Mum reaches over and turns on the lamp, encircling us in its warm, soft glow.

. . .

At four in the morning I wake with a start, my milk letting down before I consciously hear Owen cry. I don't want to wake Virginia, and I whisk, half stultified, into the study, settling Owen on my breast and myself in a low chair. The house is still, and the tiles are cold underfoot; unlike Virginia, I have no slippers. I curl my feet beneath my chair, taking care not to shift Owen lest he get any ideas about staying up. I, now, am fully awake, but the house is utterly still; it has the stillness and silence of a house full of sleep.

When Owen has settled back into the cot, bottom in the air again as he squashes his face into the mattress, I pad into the kitchen for a glass of water. The sky has that predawn false illumination, a lessening of darkness rather than the apparition of light; it is the color of faded ink. Around the room sleeping electronics show little red glowing eyes. I can't remember which way to turn the tap for cold, but the hot water takes a minute to run anyway, so it doesn't really matter; it is bone-cold as it rushes through the pipes.

For a minute I think I hear a noise, and then again: a soft groan. I walk to Virginia's closed door and listen intently, but there is silence again, and stillness. Through my mind hurtles one of those double-edged thoughts: *I should go in and see if she needs anything / If she is suffering she will want to keep it private and not be embarrassed by questions*. I wait another beat, but there is stillness, silence again, and I imagine that she was groaning in her sleep. A lifetime of reticence between us stays my hand, and I go to bed and am soon deep in sleep again.

My mother shakes my shoulder after what seems like a minute. The day has lightened, it is dawn, and I can see the dismay sketched across her face.

"Honey, I need your help," she says. "Mummy has fallen out of bed."

I am on my feet before I know it, throwing the dressing gown Virginia has lent me around my shoulders. From the other room I hear Owen stirring—he will wake soon—and we hasten around the corner of the L to get to Virginia's room. Her head and shoulders are wedged in the legs of the bedside table, and my mind flashes back immediately to that groan in the night. If she has been there all this time . . . But there is no time now to think about it—my mother is bending down to help and I do, too, automatically.

I lift one shoulder and we heave her up into sitting. She has thrown up down the front of her dress, and Mum calls an ambulance while I disappear into the en suite for a facewasher. The water runs cold, and I still cannot remember which way the heat goes, so I run into the kitchen and boil an inch of water in the kettle, soaking the cloth when the water has nearly boiled and holding it to the inside of my wrist until I think it has bearably cooled.

My mother is down on the ground with Virginia, massaging one of her legs, trying to get the feeling back into them. I pass Virginia the facewasher, and she dabs at her face and dress while I begin to massage the other leg. It is grossly swollen with fluid, the skin so dry that it seems more like a powder coating than a strong organ holding Virginia in. I push upward firmly with the palms of my hands, trying to apply only enough pressure.

"Ooh, darling, a little softer, please," she says, "that hurts."

I look at my hands, long and elegant like my mother's and Olivia's, mine good for writing, Olivia's for playing the piano. I wish more than anything that it were Claire here, not me. Virginia worked with the intellectually disabled, my mother was a special educator, but Claire has gone the furthest and works as a nurse in the neonatal intensive care unit. Her hands measure microscopic doses of medicine, clean the meconium off extremely premature babies; she would know what to do next, how to massage a swollen leg without it bringing Virginia to tears. But I think that the pain is the sensation returning, and that to help her we are inevitably going to have to hurt.

The ambulance is on its way. Mum bustles about making sure that the paramedics will have access, and tosses me a clean nightie—Virginia would die of shame to be found with vomit down her front. Some of her briskness seems to have rubbed off on me. Owen is crying; I go to comfort him, give him a biscuit and put him back in the cot, then return to where Virginia is seated on the floor, her back against a bed she will never sleep in again.

"I'm going to do this the same way I do with Owen," I tell her. "Left arm up."

Painfully, she raises her left arm, and I slip the nightie over it.

"Right arm."

When both arms are free I pull the back of the nightie over her head, folding the cloth over the vomit, and keep it there as a bib across her breasts. I settle the neck of the clean nightie around her head, then slide the soiled one out from under the clean cloth as she slips her arms into the wide holes of fresh pink cotton.

I run some water in the laundry sink, and rinse the vomit off the front of the dress, then tip in a bit of Sard and put the plug in, soaking the stain out. It doesn't occur to me, then, to put the whole thing in the bin.

The paramedics arrive as Owen's insistent babble has risen to a screech, and I recuse myself and try to keep him entertained, singing songs by rote with one ear attuned to the bedroom. Birdlife is stirring, and I take Owen out to look at the sky as Virginia is wheeled out on a gurney. She is telling the paramedics which way she wants them to drive to the hospital; she wants my mother to see the funeral parlor she has already decided upon, one she chose for its lovely view of the bay.

I bring Owen up to her cheek as she gives me a level look. I stoop down and give her a kiss, and the paramedics are ready to go, but she looks inquiringly at the baby and then breaks out into birdsong, *"Kook-kook-kook-kook-ca-ca-ca-ca-ca!"* until he raises a watery, bewildered smile. Then she is loaded into the ambulance and the doors close behind her, and my mother climbs into the front seat, and Owen and I return to the empty house.

At the funeral, grandchildren and senior citizens file into a pale pink room, taking seats on rows of chairs that have been set out neatly, the front row reserved for family. Virginia has planned a midmorning, weekday service, mostly so the more elderly of her friends and acquaintances can come. They have the look of women who have attended too many funerals, shocked that someone so much younger than them could already be gone, but fundamentally un-surprised by death.

My mother and her sisters take seats at the right side of the front row. Claire, Olivia, and I are behind them. My hands are very faintly traced with black; I managed to streak shoe polish all over my palms cleaning my shoes, and think how typical it is for me to appear before Virginia one last time in disarray. My mother is giving the eulogy, and she has anguished over it all week, reading it out for us at a family dinner the night before. We are all staying at the beach house now; during the service, Mike keeps a sleep-ing Owen company in the car.

When it is time for the eulogy, Olivia gives me a nudge and flicks her eyes over to Mum, and I nod and squeeze her hand to show that I have gotten the code. If it becomes too much for her, I will get up and read the eulogy in her place. It is not to my credit that I am good in a crisis—

some people are and some aren't, and my ability to rise to the occasion is paid for with my inability to sometimes handle the minutiae of daily life. I know that Olivia trusts in this ability, but as my mother begins to read, I see the look on her face and my heart catches in my throat. If I am asked to speak now, I am not sure whether I can.

She reads:

Not many people know that Virginia was adopted as a wee babe. Her parents, James and Lynda, were generous. They gave her a home, a private school education, and a basic framework for life. They were good people. They were also formal, and hard people, possibly a reflection of the times. My mother had to obey a complex set of rules with regard to etiquette and manners. In her family it was very much the time for children to be seen and not heard.

If she was naughty, her mother would threaten to return her to the orphanage. Maybe that was in line those days with being sold to the gypsies or bogeyman. But today as a daughter, and an early childhood educator, it breaks my heart that "little Virginia" learned to conform, or do the right thing, in order to avoid being punished.

The rest of the eulogy speaks to Virginia's strength of character: how she developed a sense of doing right for its own sake, rather than for fear of punishment; how many people she helped and championed in her work with the intellectually disabled; how missed she would be. I cannot, though, get the image of "little Virginia" out of my mind. I had known about the adoption, known about the rigidity of her adoptive parents, but when you are scared of making yourself vulnerable to somebody you lose the ability to empathize with them. Now, in the funeral home, my heart goes out to Virginia in a way that will do her no good now; it is already too late.

"During her illness we spent a lot of time together and our relationship softened and changed," my mother continues. This softening is the thing that I will come back to, the thing that I will remember; how her own daughters lost the look of wariness they sometimes wore around her; how easy it was for me to sit unguardedly and breastfeed in her big armchair. What Virginia had was presence—a mighty, pervasive charisma that she tried all her life to quash, living within the limits of what was acceptable in her own time; and that is not a crime. But it breaks my heart that she let her guard down so very late.

When I try to think about our relationship and why it was so strained, despite the love, I cannot come up with a simple illuminating example. There was never any single incident, no sharp words that bruised me so much that they stayed etched into my mind. It is simply that I, as a child, and she, as an adult, were so fundamentally at odds in the things we wanted from life that we couldn't reach out to each other in any way that the other would recognize.

And yet I know that just for a moment in time, she broke free: when she left a lonely marriage—uncaring of the opinion of neighbors, having fallen in love with Jim—and pursued that love despite the bounds of her vows, the social cost of divorce, the cost to her daughters. She threw it all away in a fit of wild longing that ultimately brought her happiness, contentment, love. When I mourn for Virginia, I mostly regret that I cannot have known this woman, who took a risk and pushed against what was expected of her, and was repaid in more riches than she could imagine, before the habits of a lifetime stilled her back into quiescence and respectability.

My son sleeps in the Princess Bed now, denuded of its frills, removed from Virginia's house, and dressed in a dinosaur Doona set that my mother went hunting for at Target. Now that Virginia has passed, my mother has become more comfortable with the idea of being called "Grannie," not wanting before to take her mother's mantle, but it is too late; she is firmly and forever "Susie" to him, his beloved Susie who picks him up and throws him around, and reads him endless stories, and takes him into the garden to help pull out the weeds.

I think of Virginia when I wear a jaunty top with nautical stripes, or when I hear a kookaburra or see an agapanthus. In her will she left her four granddaughters each a small lump sum, surprising us all, and I put mine mostly toward the debt we accrued after Owen's birth. I had enough left over to buy a new refrigerator, stainless-steel with a ten-year warranty, and, best of all, the freezer sensibly at the bottom of the machine. I felt Virginia would approve. My mother asked if I wanted anything of hers, but I didn't feel that I needed anything to hold on to, apart from the bells that she bought and played for Owen. Virginia herself passed down a big, soft cotton scarf, cream-and-brown paisley with a pea-soup-green border. It is beautiful, and I wrap it around my head on days when I don't want to wash my hair, trusting in its beauty to disguise my scruffiness and fatigue.

With my hair pulled up, I look less like Virginia than usual; the strong Hungarian planes of my brow and nose seem to come to the fore. Sometimes I get compliments on the street, most often from the florist; sometimes a passing woman catches the corner of my eye, a woman with a dark crisp bob, or large pearls and a certain set of the mouth, and for a minute Virginia is with me, just for a moment and always on the move. Then she is gone and I continue on my way, heading down the street for a coffee with Mum, and safe in the knowledge that she will never, ever die.

WALKING

EVERY MORNING, my father goes for an hour's walk before work. This is the ritual that starts the day. When I come down to the kitchen for breakfast he is just getting home, and the dog precedes him through the door, pattering around, looking for a sunny patch, while my dad dumps the shrink-wrapped tube of the newspaper on the kitchen table. Often it is damp with condensation, but when I peel the wrapping off, the newsprint itself is dry.

Depending on the season, my sisters and I wear identical pale blue knee socks with our school uniforms, or itchy, dark gray tights. Dad's early-morning outfit is unvaried; tracksuit pants, a T-shirt, sneakers, and a jumper tied around his waist, disguising or reinforcing the back brace he wears on cold mornings. His back injury is one of the reasons for his walking, and for the careful, constant stretches he does. After dinner, he leaves the table and rolls his knees from side to side upon the floor.

As a child, I have no clear idea of what a disk is, or what it means to "slip" one or two or three. In my mind, my father's spine is like a Jenga tower, with pieces sticking out precipitously, ready to bring the entire structure down. In fact, his spine is not too dissimilar now to a stack of blocks—bone on bone with nothing to cushion each vertebra. He teases his mother about the fact that she is shrinking, but he is not as tall as he was.

Every now and then, on a High Holiday or when someone has died, my father gets up early to accompany his father to shul, walking there, of course, because on these occasions you don't drive. I don't know what kind of tricky political maneuvering has gotten him to this point, or what strings have been pulled, but these mornings come as a kind of détente in an ongoing tussle over Dad's lack of faith. He himself disclaimed religion years and years ago, but neither of his parents really accept that he no longer believes in God; or if they do, they believe that his defection is too late; he has already been bar mitzvahed, and that is that.

My dad keeps a few yarmulkes in a drawer in the hallway console, between misplaced golf tees and a set of spare keys. When I accompany my grandmother, Nagyi, to shul myself on odd occasions, I sit with her on the women's balcony, something that must have been brought over from the old country, because in the early '90s, who segregates men and women? Only the most conservative, but I don't have any idea of the fault lines yet between Orthodox and Progressive, Hasidic and Reform. In my grandparents' neighborhood, girls wear wigs and long black skirts, but Nagyi disdains them for their showiness. There are ways and ways to be a good conservative Jew.

On High Holidays, the main ways are prayer and food. Inevitably we three girls will arrive tetchy from being bundled into our "good" clothes and then sitting around afraid to mark them. We have Peter Pan collars edged with lace, and large velvet headbands holding back our glossy hair. We are keyed up, too, with the awareness of something special happening, but unable to read all the currents of the evening, the ebbs and flows.

In the kitchen Nagyi gossips with a Hungarian woman she will have hired for the evening, though it seems to save her little work. We barely see her as she hovers between the kitchen and the formal dining room, with its dark green flocked wallpaper, polished dark wood, crisp white linen. Dinner, in the Hungarian tradition, starts with a bowl of soup, which I love—Nagyi's chicken soup, which sets to a kind of gel when it cools. There is a ritual aspect to this first course; bowls are brought out two by two on a wooden tray, and it feels like a milestone the year that I am trusted to carry it and not spill a drop.

Depending on the holiday, Papa's intonement of Hebrew is either brief or on-and-on-and-on. Dad jokes that all Jewish holidays boil down to "They tried to kill us, they failed, let's eat!" but I scrupulously study the English text in the Haggadah, trying to make sense of it, or at least match the English words to the Hebrew rhythm. Some aspect of me feels that I ought to find this language resonant, or at least imbued with meaning, but it goes over my head, and the meal is reduced to a pantomime. We play a children's pantomime, too, toward the end, hiding a piece of matzo for my grandfather to studiously not find, and bargaining its release for a net of gold chocolate coins.

At some point I ask Dad why he left the shul, and he tells it very simply: that he went every Saturday until he was seventeen years old, when he raised a scriptural question from the day's sermon with his father; that Papa told him very firmly not to question the rabbi, and since that point my father has had no faith. There is a horror around that quashing of spirit that is too great for my child's mind to take in, and I put it away, unaware that it has tangled in my mind with a budding supposition—that Jews can get in trouble if they ask too many questions.

Questions are my lifeblood; I cannot live without them. As my legs grow longer I like to join Dad in the morning, prowling the suburbs before the sun comes up. It takes me a while to wake up all the way, but I love the feeling of the wind brisking up my cheeks as we cross the bridge into Richmond. As we head over the river we can see rowers out in pairs or single sculls, seagulls perched on the garbage traps, long snaky strands of gold light rippling with the flow of the water.

Often we walk in silence, the dog trotting at my father's side. The sky turns pink and crisp in the autumn, and balloons go up over the city. When we talk, I bounce my newly forming philosophical quandaries off my father, who enjoys them. "How do I know that the color *I* see as green is the same color that *you* see as green?" I ask, and for the next twenty minutes we are down a path that is composed half of classical philosophies of subjectivity, and half of how the eye actually perceives color as a lens. It amazes me that there are wavelengths of light—all around me and going *through* me—that I cannot detect at all.

Every term, we carry our school reports to our grandparents' house, and they read over them and congratulate us, and my grandfather solemnly hands to each of us an envelope of cash. The money embarrasses me, but the pride I enjoy. I know how much it means to him to see us do well; he left school at fourteen himself, to help his parents in their shop, in the country town my grandmother would later live in and loathe. He was the second eldest, and survived the Holocaust with five of his siblings—six out of nine. They were the largest group of siblings to survive; I think there is a certificate somewhere.

The fact of this is somewhere in the background, also squashed, also repressed. When I come across Jewish children in *When Hitler Stole Pink Rabbit* or *Number the Stars*, I am careful not to invest too much of myself into them. It is easier to be Laura Ingalls Wilder or Emily of New Moon, or Jo March, with her independence and her comically small head. I tear through everything the junior school library has to offer, then get special permission to visit the senior school library for books.

Nagyi and Papa come to our end-of-year assemblies; they are faithful attendees of our recitals and ballet concerts. Dad watches the unbending of his father with astonishment. When I miss a mark in a spelling test, he shakes his head with mock dismay.

"You know when I was your age, if I brought home a test with a mark of ninety-six, my father would say, 'What happened to the other four points?'"

I laugh, trying not to show how much I mind those few missed marks. I hear the conversations between my teachers, and I know that some of the work I am given is different, harder. The word *potential* is used cautiously; I begin to realize that I have a great deal of potential. But the thinly veiled excitement behind the phrase is a compliment I haven't yet earned. I am expected to *do* something with this potential; I am supposed to live up to it; there is no telling how far I will go.

My parents pick up on and try to assuage my anxiety. "I don't care if you want to be a garbage collector," says Dad, "just as long as you are the best garbage collector you can be."

Later I find that this is a mantra in all migrant households, and one that my friends trot out when we are telling the stories of where we came from. *The best you can be* echoes around the back of my skull, a lone refrain until

I abandon my homework one night as mostly done, good enough. Dad looks at me over the top of his newspaper when I say as much out loud.

"There is no such thing," he says, "as 'good enough.'"

My mother is horrified to overhear this, but Dad looks me in the eye, and I know exactly what he means.

The school that my sisters and I attend is called Barbreck, the junior school sister of a single-sex private institution. It doesn't occur to me to find a school comprising only women and girls odd; at home Dad often groans jokingly of being outnumbered, though he wanted six girls initially. I am comfortable in the presence of women and girls. The boys I know are fun, but not in the inner circle.

We are here in part because of my mother's hairy legs. As a teenage girl, she tells me later, she deliberately lagged to the back of cross-country running groups so that the older boys would not see her legs. She didn't want us ever not to be swift; she didn't want us to sabotage our chances, to feel the shame of exposure. She tells me about the incinerators in the girls' toilets at her senior school; how girls were required to burn their bulky sanitary pads, and any girl bleeding was identifiable from the plume of smoke emerging above her toilet stall, announcing her like the election of a new pope. Later, on her teaching rounds, she gritted her teeth as boys pushed their way to the new computers at the expense of their female peers, and were rewarded with attention and opportunity for it.

Barbreck is warm and kind and faithfully ambitious. It is the '90s, and our mothers have been chipping away at the glass ceiling, trying to keep splinters of glass out of their perms. One year we host an "astronaut-in-residence," Dr. Rhea Seddon, a brilliant physician, one of the first women to go to space. She teaches science in the senior school and appears at our assemblies, where we regard her with awe. Blond and trim and indefinably American, she embodies something toward which our tiny hearts yearn. We can do anything, we are told, if only we believe in ourselves, and work hard, and never let anyone make us think that we are not as good as men.

That we can have and be anything we want is borne out by our parents, who, if they are not old money, are migrants or the children of migrants; our mothers and fathers, but mostly our fathers, started out with nothing, and look at them now. In the playground there is no feeling of racial consciousness; though I don't know the term *model minority* yet, that is what we are, we migrant daughters of Jewish and Chinese and Indian doctors and lawyers.

My race education is of its place and time, which will make me blush as an adult when I understand what this means. I am sure we do learn about Indigenous Australians, whom we call Aborigines, sometime during primary school; I am sure that I make a poster presentation. I know that at some point we learn about bush tucker, and place tiny native-pepper berries on our tongues, and squirm and giggle at the thought of eating witchetty grubs. We all have enough food at home; we cannot imagine that anyone, by necessity or choice, would eat a bug.

We also learn that Captain Cook "discovered" Australia in 1770, that he and Joseph Banks staked a claim on Botany Bay and then the nation began; that from then on colonies sprang up, and convicts worked through their indenture, and the Gold Rush brought prosperity, and sheep and wheat and opals brought even more. We do not learn about the Frontier Wars, or if we do, they are not named as such, and the losses of life are downplayed. If we learn about the referendum to repeal Section 127 of the Constitution, reading *In reckoning the numbers of the people of the Commonwealth, or of a State or other part of the Commonwealth, aboriginal natives shall not be counted*, it is as a footnote to history, not something that I, or anyone else, has ever made a diorama about.

My family and I move to a Victorian dollhouse closer to our school. I have the smallest bedroom, a hideaway hole—I have always loved nooks. It overlooks the back stairs down to the garden, their iron railing covered in passion-fruit vine. I fall asleep to the sound of laundry in the washing machine in the room below: *swish swish swish*. It is almost like hearing the ocean. My sister has brought her rabbits, but there are foxes in this neighborhood, and at some point the rabbits vanish beneath the fence.

There is a deep armchair under the window in Dad's study, and this is where I spend most of my afternoons, especially as the weather turns chill. There is less time now for dreaming, and less for reading, at least reading for pleasure. School is starting to crowd in, filling my time with quadratic equations, and the altitude of Mount Saint Helens, and the poetry of Gwen Harwood, which I adore.

There is also, pervasively, the Holocaust. It seems to permeate the entirety of our classes for a term, in History and in English, as the scale of World War II is pressed upon us again and again. We read Livia Bitton-Jackson's book *Elli*, and it doesn't escape me that Elli's surname is the same as mine; that we are both fourteen. I read it once, put it down, and move on to other things. I don't want to dwell on this book, or on the immensity of its subject.

One image sticks with me vividly, though: girls marching naked toward Auschwitz, one of them bleeding freely down her thighs, and Elli's sudden realization that she might one day be as embarrassed and exposed as that. In a girls' school, pads and tampons are batted around the bathrooms with nonchalance. They are wrapped in bright colors, and girls read out the trivia printed on their hygiene stickers from behind the stall doors.

The girls who are not the daughters of migrants have long sleek ponytails and suntanned legs. A few years earlier, they passed around a copy of *Bridge to Terebithia*, highly prized because it made them cry *so* much. It is not a crime to be sentimental, but when we are given a creative writing exercise—to produce an account of life in Auschwitz and Dachau—I feel my gorge rising on a hot tide of panic. I do not have the language to explain, even to myself, how sick I feel about these girls indulging in the *so sad* sadness of life within a camp, even in fiction, even for a minute.

I think about writing a letter to my teacher explaining this, but I don't. It doesn't occur to me to simply not do the work; I am too much of a Goody Two-shoes, a perfect student, a suck. And I know that I will have to face what happened in Hungary and Germany and Poland at some point, so I tell myself I am being mature and write the piece. And I get full marks, and I do not wallow and I do not flinch. But later, when I have learned the language of *appropriation* and *thanatourism* and the concept of *trauma porn*, I will wish that I had not been such a coward, and that instead I had simply told my English teacher to fuck off.

More and more I come to value the time spent walking in the morning before school. At sixteen I am in my final year of school, and so, unlike my friends, I don't rush out and get my license straightaway. The thought of learning to drive, on top of the schoolwork that is piling up, feels like too much pressure, too much stress.

I am still intent on following my father, who is a dentist, into some kind of medical field, preferably surgery—from a young age I have been fascinated with the workings of the body—and so I immerse myself in chemistry and mathematical methods, the latter of which I loathe. I like chemistry for its acceptance of ambiguity, its stoichiometric equations that acknowledge that no state of matter is ever truly fixed, and its insight into organisms, their flux and their flow. I love reading about how carbohydrates break down in the stomach, and drawing the branching-out molecules of various structures of fat.

The open-and-closed fixity of math depresses me, sparking the beginnings of panic. I know that somewhere much more advanced in the field a redeeming openness is possible, but I can't get my feet to stay on the lowest rungs or grasp the simplest logics. My dreams are filled with antidifferential equations that are insoluble, as they seem in waking life. I send my brain out probing for answers, and the best I can do is find an answer that *feels* right; I work backward from the area I think the answer resides, and when I am right I am still wrong because I cannot show my work.

Because I have taken the year-twelve literature units already, I am allowed to enroll in an extension program at the university, claiming the credit toward my VCE and also, somehow, toward my first year in arts if I enroll in that degree. When the bell rings I fly out of the classroom and toward the toilets, stripping off my gray sack of a school uniform and stuffing myself into jeans and thick jumpers, yanking the elastic out of my hair and shaking it free. If I race down the hill I can catch the train into the city, then the tram to uni, and be in Parkville by the time lectures start at 4:15 p.m.

At university, I am giddy with release; if I venture an opinion, someone else will pick it up and tease it apart, or rebut it, and then we will be in full swing, raised voices, debating fiercely. In lectures I learn about Habermas and

Foucault, about performativity and scansion and the Death of the Author and how to take good notes. When I join the others for a drink at the university bar, nobody asks me for ID. I get used to drinking beer that tastes of wet carpet; it is heavy on the belly, but cheap.

Our early-morning walks take us past a little row of shops, where Dad and I slow our pace to navigate around the café tables that have been placed out for the early rush and shoppers coming out of the bakery clutching loaves of bread. A few years of after-school work at Bakers Delight have inured me to the smell of hot bread in the morning; it is a smell I miss, a comfort smell. At one shop front I sneak a quick glance at a pair of shoes in the window. They are flat sandals with an open back, with metal hoops and disks of black leather arcing over the top of the foot. They look like something Kate Bush would wear.

When I get my results, I let out a whoop, and then sit for a moment, looking at the computer screen. I have slept until noon to safely ignore the phone calls of curious family, and I know that my parents must be dying of tension in the other room, where they are respecting my distance while I find out whether or not I've got the marks I need. I have missed out on a place in medicine by one point, but I feel curiously light having had the decision made for me, and deeply content about my impending entry into arts.

I tell my parents my score, and they hug me and ring my grandparents, and later in the day Dad presents me with a box. In it are the Kate Bush shoes. I know that secretly he would like to mark the occasion by giving me a car, but these shoes are much, much dearer to me. I hadn't realized that he'd been watching each morning when I paused at the shopwindow to admire them and say hello.

In the first year of my arts degree, uniforms left behind forever, an older girl in my art history class takes me under her wing, and my life opens up in a way I have longed for, inchoately, for as long as I have known. Summer evenings pass in cheap apartments above shops, playing records on a machine bought at Vinnies and smoking on the roof, or in tiny paved back gardens, sitting on upturned milk crates between the back door and the dunny. I go to a fancy-dress party dressed as Annie Hall and fall in love with a lean, dark-haired boy in the corner, his brown eyes glowing over the light of his cigarette. I leave our conversation to go to the loo, unclipping my father's borrowed suspenders.

"Absolutely not," my friend hisses while I'm away. "She's seventeen years old." But a year later I am half living at his house, waking up lazily and putting the stovetop espresso on while his housemates go to Tabet's for cheese-and-spinach pies. We watch *Betty Blue* and play backgammon in the morning, clean up haphazardly, take cups of tea out into the backyard with the newspaper or an old copy of *Heat*. When his Deleuze reading group comes over, I head out the back and read fashion magazines. I already know my position on Deleuze.

It is here that I read *Monkey Grip* for the first time, and feel a faint marvel of clairsentience at Helen Garner's prose. So I haven't dreamed up this life out of whole cloth; it exists, it has existed before me and without me, and was waiting for me to come and inhabit it, to walk the very same streets I am now walking, and argue over ethics and love and sex, and obsessively *write*. I curl up on Tom's ratty old couch with my feet in a pair of his socks, the heels coming up past the back of my ankles, and scrawl poems on the backs of old envelopes as my mind flies far above the plum trees and the washing line.

As I am growing older, my grandparents grow older, too. For years Nagyi has been abetting Papa as he slowly declines into what will be confirmed, later, as dementia. She is so canny, and her personality so forceful, that if any of us suspect that she is covering for him, we keep it to ourselves. The role of neurotic, fussy Jewish mother—and grandmother—is culturally prevalent; she leans into it hard. Another joke of my father's: "A Jewish mother gives her son two ties for his birthday. He comes down to breakfast the next day wearing one of them and she says, 'What, you didn't like the other one?'"

At Seder we still play out the ritual of hiding the matzo, though in increasingly obvious hiding places, and increasingly it becomes obvious that he genuinely cannot find it. We all love this man: the strength of his back, his too-strong hands, his ability to fold laundry impeccably, a relic of his days in *schmatte*. I love him achingly, although for a long time now I have understood the undercurrents of earlier years; my mother's tension headaches; the things that were said when my father married out. When my mother offered to convert, Dad threw a fit; his parents would accept her as she was, or not at all. But it put us, as children, in a precarious situation.

Papa's memories, long repressed, begin to come to the surface. Nagyi has made an oral history for a friend's daughter's PhD, but now I steel myself to interview her, for my first book chapter, a published work; I think, mistakenly, that I can do the work of honoring this chapter of her life in five thousand words, over two afternoons. I want it out of my system, where it has taken up residence like a ghost. It is not my story; but it is in my body, it is in my blood.

Nagyi's sister Anne joins us, and the two of them prompt each other, speaking rapidly in Magyar. What I learn has already come out in dribs and drabs, in offhand comments over the years. That the bodies were piled so high that after a while these piles began to seem ordinary. That they stitched gold stars to their lapels and slept bone-weary and cold on cots in the "good" ghetto, and were not lined up and shot into the Danube, and were not raped, they stress, not by the Hungarians, not by the Germans, and not by the Americans, who, in their jubilation and reckless-ness, may have been the cruelest of all.

Papa, though, has never spoken of the war. I only have the barest outlines: a Russian labor camp; the fact that his sister died in Auschwitz, that he has never said her name. He is gentle with our dog, but gets skittish when he hears him growling; I see him cringe almost imperceptibly, a reflex that goes against everything he knows about Alex's fierce allegiance to all members of our family. A labor camp, dogs, and the fact that there are virtually no Jews left in Kisvárda today; these are the dots I try not to connect.

My parents help renovate the bathroom of my grandparents' house, taking out the deep bath and installing a shower with room for a chair, and handrails. The deep blue hexagonal tiles, in a pattern I have always loved, are ripped up to show a wound where the bath once was. A long stretch of fresh grout smooths over this edge, but it is the beginning of change. I can't remember now if there was a fall; it seems likely that there was. By the time I am in my second year of university, Papa is in a hospital bed, and we are gathered around, waiting.

My life out in the world is everything I want it to be, but sometimes my child self catches up to me, anxious, nauseous, wanting so badly to please. I try to ignore this sense of being doubled, being always followed by a sadness I can't explain. If my childhood was happy, and it so very often was, then how did the sadness get in?

There is no room in the story of a richly nourished and nurtured childhood for this sadness. There is no explaining why, even as a very young child, I am sometimes paralyzed in the night by a wash of loneliness so powerful that by morning I have buried it deep within me. The child psychologists I see, usually for only three or four sessions and only every two or three years, find nothing wrong with me other than a tendency to worry and the usual signs of giftedness. I am enrolled in extension programs, my parents hoping, I think, to burn off some of this anxiety through intellectual stimulation, in the same way puppies exhaust themselves into contentedness at the dog park.

Nobody at this time mentions the concept of intergenerational trauma, much less epigenetic history. Somewhere in California, Mike's father is working on the supercomputer that will finally map the genome. DNA is an exciting new frontier, but its applications are still thought of as physical, not psychological. It is only as an adult that I encounter the idea of histones—those protective, elegant proteins cushioning the gene—and the research that demonstrates methylation and histone modification altering the behavior and memory of laboratory mice.

There is a famous experiment involving mice that were trained to fear the scent of acetophenone, a compound associated with the smell of cherries, by being given electric shocks. Their pups and even their grandpups were introduced to this smell after they were born, and showed a marked trauma reaction, having never experienced an electric shock or smelled or seen a cherry. I think about this a lot.

In human behavioral studies, the children and grandchildren of Holocaust survivors—the largest study population easily available to Western researchers—have been found to be demonstrably more resilient or, on the contrary, more vulnerable to stress than others. There is "a chemical coating upon [our] chromosomes, which would represent a kind of biological memory of what the parents experienced,"[1] one researcher writes, and I wonder again at this doubling: What makes some become more resilient, some less?

I do not tell any of my child psychologists about the fact that I see ghosts; they disappear in the daytime, and I feel foolish for having believed in them. But sometimes late at night, in the space between waking and sleeping, I am seized with fear, terrified to move my arms or legs; my skin becomes hot, my heart beats erratically, and I become hypervigilant, because I am sure that I can feel a cool breeze on my face, or a presence in the room. It is not sleep paralysis, which I learn about later, because I *can* move my limbs, I am simply too scared to, and my mouth tastes like bitter almonds as the fear slowly ebbs away.

In my late teens there are days when I can barely leave the house for thinking about the world; days when I stand paralyzed in the kitchen doorway for half an hour, unable to eat because the choice between toast and muesli is fraught, and something catastrophic will happen if I'm wrong. I no longer open the mail and the electricity to our sharehouse is cut off; the ghosts have become internalized now, they are dybbukim. I can no longer see them, but they still have the terrifying ability to grab me, without warning, and hold me in stasis.

I am eighteen, nineteen, twenty, and I have still not

learned to drive. My grandmother learned at the age of forty-six, I tell myself, there is no rush, I have plenty of time. On my long legs I stalk vast swaths of the inner north, trying to exhaust myself on the nights I cannot sleep. The truth is I am petrified of getting behind the wheel; of the strength and power of a ton of metal beneath the touch of my hands and feet, of the compulsion I can feel when I'm only *imagining* driving to swing the wheel, drive too fast, cause a crash deliberately. I am not safe and I can't feel safe. And so the soles of my feet get worn and tough, pacing and mapping the suburbs under dim electric lights.

To my grandfather, education is a priority above nearly everything else. Part of it, I am sure, comes from the fact that, due to his family's poverty, he never got to pursue a higher education. My grandmother, living in Budapest, could have afforded it, but was barred of course, because she was a Jew. Unable to go to university, she trained as a beautician instead, something that probably saved them from starvation under Communism later; there was no state-affiliated cosmetology, so her small private business was allowed to stay open, half sanctioned, flying beneath the radar.

Part of the thirst for knowledge undoubtedly comes, too, from the Jewish requirement to study and learn from the Torah; from the long, five-thousand-year-rich Jewish oral-history tradition that kept the faith alive under multiple occupancies, Europe and Africa over. I have always liked this, from Philo of Alexandria in the first century AD:

> Since the Jews esteem their laws as divine
> revelations, and are instructed in the knowledge
> of them from their earliest youth, they bear
> the image of the law in their souls.

Knowledge, for the Jew, is spiritual; *hunger* for knowledge is spiritual. This is as close to any religious tenet that I absolutely believe.

In fact, the simplest explanation is probably the ghetto reason: education is something that *nobody can take away from you*. It is part of basic human dignity to keep a storehouse of truths and stories in some part of your psyche, or soul if you believe you have one; degradation that is imposed from the outside can be borne as long as you know who you are.

But there is knowledge and there is knowledge. It is true that some things seem permanently etched somewhere inside me, often forgotten for years and then retrieved out of nowhere: the sound of Nina Simone singing "Break Down and Let It All Out"; the fairy tales I absently tell Owen; my father's shoelaces, looping around each other as Olivia stealthily ties them together at his feet. He is sitting in his spot on the old brown leather couch, its arm worn thin over a deadly wooden block that is ready to catch you on the side of the hip as you fling yourself into the chair. The footy is on and Dad is reading a newspaper—he claims he can read and watch at the same time. At his right is a glass of scotch and an opaque white plastic Tupperware container, a cylinder that is labeled with the word ALMONDS in text that is wearing faint. Olivia ties his shoelaces together and then sneaks off, holding her mirth in, as one of us other girls flops across Dad's shoulder and reaches for the remote.

I can remember this; it is vivid and clear as day, but my brain is already busy working, dismantling the memory, peopling it with alternating sisters or changing out clothes. Is it the mustard or the red-and-blue-striped jumper he is wearing? Is Alex, our beautiful big schnauzer, flopped at his feet? And what is it he's shouting at the television? It is probably a variant of "Round the neck!" or "Come on, umpire!" or "That's gotta be fifty!"—phrases of pure ocker that slip out from time to time from a place of deep assimilation.

It always makes me laugh to hear them, though I know he has earned the right to call the umpire a bloody white maggot. When he stands around the barbecue with my mother's brothers-in-law and says things like "Strewth!" and "Kenoath!" I know he is hamming it up, but it is also a proof of something: affection and warmth that broaches difference; a shibboleth of belonging.

I do not want to take these things away from him. I can feel my mind always picking away at something, unbuilding and reconstructing it. It is the only way I know. *Knowledge* for me does not mean *facts*, and a thing is never done and dusted, and constantly questioning is exhausting, but I cannot turn my mind off. I am as tiny as a quark or an atom; if something appears to be solid, I still slip right through it, and it is hard to settle comfortably into ever staying in one place.

. . .

It doesn't escape my attention that everyone in *Monkey Grip* is white, or that at the parties I go to, few people didn't go to private school. We may have pissed off away from the values of our parents, but we are still, inescapably, products of our environments.

I settle down to write my thesis and try to come to grips with some of it, the morass of existence, searching the work of four poets for some link between the violence in their work, the fractures of their language, and their attitude to the land for some clue that will prove illuminating, and settle some of my anxieties. I am trying to resolve the settler-colonial problem, by myself, in a poetry thesis that no one will read. The poets I examine are settler-colonial or migrant; including Indigenous poetries will blow out my word limit by three or four times, but I still loathe myself for this exclusion.

When I visit my parents' house my dad and I resume our conversations, which over the years have become arguments, pitched battles, as I move away from his particular worldview. In moments of quiet, we are still each other's best friends. Walking together, sitting and reading, there is a current flowing between us that comes of a mutual love and understanding of who we are aside from our thoughts.

But neither of us is the kind to bite their tongue, and the arguments, left off, will always be resumed. He thinks I am a Pinko-Commie-Greenie bleeding heart, and I say of course I am, that that is the heart's function, to pump blood, to power the whole machine through its bleeding. He baits me persistently, and my sisters sink into their chairs as we begin, quietly at first and then with raised voices, to go over and over ground that neither of us will cede.

What infuriates me the most about these debates is that I can never seem to win. My father, with his scientist's ability to learn by rote, has a vast storehouse of facts that sound extremely dubious but that I can't refute with analysis, which is my strongest tool; his reach is vast, there are statistics to back up everything. I still cannot memorize a phone number, or quickly add up a bill. I get lost amid a wash of numbers I am sure are being construed wrongly, and cannot seem to right them.

I know, intellectually, that it is better to be stymied at every turn by someone you love and respect than by someone you loathe and fear. There is never any nastiness in these arguments, but still they get beneath my skin.

"Look," my dad says, "there have always been fluctuations in climate. Look at the Ice Age. When you say 'the hottest June' on record, yeah, well, we've only been keeping records for a hundred years! It's hubris to believe that humans can change the climate."

"Jesus! It's hubris to believe we haven't!"

When I get to the point of hollering, my mum steps in. *This isn't rhetorical*, I think wildly, *this is really happening*. I cannot stop thinking about the melting ice caps, or a teenager standing in line in the hot sun on Nauru, waiting for hours for a single tampon while the blood trickles down her leg. My grandparents walking through a field to get to the border, bribing a Russian guard in the dead of night.

One of my father's mantras is "There are no new jokes, just new audiences." Another is "Never spoil a good story with the truth." The two of them, together, seem to form an unassailable fortress. Another favorite saying, when we were children, and blocking the television: "Honey, you're a pain, but not a pane of glass." Sometimes at dinner I *do* feel like a pane of glass. The things that are so self-evident to me, the things I fight for, believe to be compellingly true, fade away to hazy transparency at his unwillingness to budge.

It is not just the climate, it is not just asylum seekers, it is not just gay marriage—for which Dad deploys reasoned and sensible arguments based on respecting the official process by which he himself came as a refugee, and for further entrenching a division of church and state. I can hurl ideology at my father as much as I want, but it won't sway him over, and I cannot resolve the party lines that are drawn within my body, through the fact of my being.

It is the whiteness, precarious and volatile. It is the Jewishness, to which I am officially denied a claim but with which I identify so strongly, in memory and in blood. It is the fact of my dad having married out, having never taught me Magyar, though I pestered him to as a child. It is the fact of an assimilation so rapid and successful that within a generation, for the most part, we have forgotten that Ashkenazi Jews ever were anything but white. In America and Australia and Britain, we have left behind the fact of being "ethnic," blending so successfully with the general population that we are no more noticeable than flies.

I read about William Cooper in one of Gary Foley's papers,[2] a historical figure I had never heard of before; a Yorta Yorta man who saw Europe's Jews as kindred:

> In November 1938, throughout Germany a major Nazi pogrom was conducted against the Jewish community. This notorious event was dubbed *kristallnacht* and signalled a dramatic upsurge of violence, intimidation and persecution of Germany's Jewish population. Less than one month later, on December 6th 1938, on the other side of the world, a Victorian Aboriginal man, William Cooper, led a deputation of Kooris from the Australian Aborigines League, in a visit to the German Consulate in Melbourne where they attempted to present a resolution "condemning the persecution of Jews and Christians in Germany." The Consul-General, Dr. R.W. Drechsler, refused them admittance.

Like the Jews, Indigenous Australians were rounded up, incarcerated, subjected to eugenic experimentation— though the latter came, for Indigenous people, not at the hands of a single demonic figure like Mengele, but through a state-sponsored program of child removal designed to rescue the light-skinned and breed out the rest. Foley writes:

> It is probable that the ironies of the deputation's visit to the German Consulate were part of the group's strategy to draw attention to the similarities between what was happening in Germany and how Aborigines were being dealt with in Australia. If that was the case it must be said that their remarkable action achieved little in mobilising the conscience of mainstream Australia either in terms of the situation of Germany's Jews or that of Aboriginal Australia. Indeed, their gesture has been almost completely forgotten in Australian history.

In the way in which you learn about something for the first time, only to have it arise again almost immediately, I hear through a Jewish friend about a playwright, Elise Hearst, who is writing about this incident. It is being co-authored by one of Cooper's descendants, Andrea James, and swiftly turns from a period piece to a metafiction; the threads are so entangled between James and Hearst, and the relationship so complex, that the two women wind up onstage as actors, reenacting the fraught lines between them; their bloodlines, the history of their ancestors, the stories they carry in their skin.

When the play is staged, I cannot make it, but I listen

to excerpts on the radio thirstily. I have never heard anything like this before, and yet it seems deeply familiar, as though dredged out of my body and my brain. It is comic, it can't help being comic, as when Andrea, lightly fictionalized, confronts Elise about the fact that a white actor is playing a Tamil ancestor:

> **ANDREA:** First all you white people nearly exterminate us, then when there are virtually no roles left for black people on stage and TV, you want to take our roles, too!
>
> **ELISE:** I'm not a white person!
>
> **ANDREA:** Aren't you?
>
> **ELISE:** No! I'm Jewish, I didn't do that stuff to your people. In fact I empathize with your suffering. Didn't you see me in that last scene getting hurled into a garage, beaten and degraded?[3]

I'm not a white person. Aren't you? In Hungary, where István the First declared that to become Catholic was to become part of Europe, and where Jews and pagans were ostracized, uncoupled from national identity by their refusal to convert, we weren't white; in the beginning decades of the twentieth century, where race and ethnicity were entangled in a hundred different ways, we weren't white. Under Hitler's fictitious and cynical categorizations of the Jews as a race, bound by eugenic claims that would be "substantiated" in horror, we weren't Aryan, we weren't citizen, we weren't white.

But when the boat carrying my grandparents and my father crossed the equator, and the hemispheres shifted beneath the waves, a transmutation took place, one that rippled like a tide from the banks of Australia's shores and back toward them again: "not-white" became, in policy and thought, a less pressing category than "not-black." In this way we took our assimilation from visible contrast to a much, much darker race, one that did not yet have full recognition under the law, as European émigrés immediately were granted. To be European became geographic, not ideological; almost as soon as we stepped upon the shores, we became cosmopolitan and the persecution ceased.

If white guilt, as Eula Biss writes,[4] stems from the same root as white debt, then the debt I think about is not the small one: the debt we owe William Cooper for extending us the recognition of our humanity, when he himself was denied it by government, was not even let into the building to present his petition, in fact. What I think about is the far, far greater indebtedness we bear, as Ashkenazis, to all of those with black and brown and Asian skins. Because whether we think of ourselves as white or not, and whether or not we desire the privileges and protections of that whiteness, we could only have obtained its protections while the nation's punitive racial agenda was bearing down elsewhere.

The small debt, to an extent, has been repaid. There is

a history of Jewish involvement in the fight for Indigenous rights of which we can justly be proud. But I flinch when I think of the thousands of years for which the Jews existed successfully as a diaspora, and the ease by which that diaspora has displaced others in order to survive, not heeding, or deliberately repressing, the damage. To open our *schmatte* factories and to educate our children, to live safely without fear of persecution, we have taken land that is not ours to take, broken spiritual ties, severed connections to country that can never be restored.

And whether or not it was done in innocence, it makes me burn with shame. I carry that shame in my body, next to my father's stroppy agnosticism and my grandmother's survivor's guilt. I feel it when I think of everything I have gained from assimilation, and everything others have lost. It is the question beneath the question, a plea for absolution. *I empathize with your suffering. Didn't you see me suffering, too?*

To walk is to wander, and that is something we are possibly cursed with. There is a flower known as the Wandering Jew, and this is the way it grows: rapidly, the legs outstripping the leaves, so that pinching it back almost annually is the only way to keep it from death.

The Wandering Jew is a flower, but he is also a person, condemned to walk the earth until Christ rises again. He is a bogeyman of medieval literature, a cautionary tale—for taunting Christ on the cross he will never settle again. For this act, or for the act of putting Christ to death, we have become dispersed, scattered across the globe. Quietly, we have traveled everywhere, learned all languages, learned to keep our customs in secret and our bodies out of danger.

That Jews are reputed to be neurotic, possibly epigenetically, that we are paranoid, that we suffer from persecution complexes, is easy to understand. We have always packed up quietly and left in the night, melting away into the darkness before the bread has had a chance to rise.

But the paranoia cuts both ways. Because of our rapid assimilation, because of our ability to mimic and impersonate—the Jews in Hollywood, the Jews in comedy—we could be anyone, anywhere. At the root of countless conspiracy theories we are there, secretly, controlling the media or America or the banks. Like a potato creeper taken for jasmine, or a tomato mischaracterized as a vegetable when really it is a fruit; to be Jewish is to be a simulacrum, so near to the thing itself that you are indistinguishable until somebody looks too close.

In the same way, as I become an adult, I hide my illness almost perfectly well. I attend nearly every class, manage to corral my anxiety into essay writing, never think to ask for special consideration at the university, even when I do spend half the week unable to get out of bed. My illness comes in fits and starts, and sometimes I am so radiantly healthy, and dance at parties, and write so persuasively that I manage to convince myself that what I am experiencing is just creative temperament; that it is romantic, and that all great artists suffer. This doesn't change the fact that when I am suffering I can barely read a magazine, let alone write a poem, but it does allow me to feel normal, feel healthy, turn my back on the fact of being debilitated.

For most of my life I am very, very good at passing.

After Owen is born, and as I sink swiftly into depression, and am no longer fooling anybody, I walk all over Footscray, pushing the baby and narrating my steps, as suggested by the hospital psychologist; it is supposed to ground you to say the things you are doing at the moment that you are doing them, to narrow your scope to the immediacy of voice and breath. What I think about instead is the land as it must have been just a whisper ago, before the boat carrying my father arrived, before the boat carrying my mother's ancestors arrived. I wonder what songlines[5] I am tracing as I walk around the river, comforting myself with the fact that I am not fit to carry them anyway, and envy the pakeha women at the park, white New Zealanders, for their casual naming of things to their children: *paihamu*, *rakiraki*, *kikorangi*.

I pace the river alone in part because I have no mother's group. When Owen is born, I attend fortnightly health checks with the maternal and child health nurse, making sure that he is okay, although increasingly she turns her attention toward me, using the Edinburgh Postnatal Depression Scale (EPDS), a set of screening questions that gives a rudimentary idea of whether a patient is suffering or not.

The nurse apologizes for the fact that there is no mother's group currently available, though I have no actual desire to attend one.

"Usually we would be able to put you in touch with some new mums in your suburb," she says, "but there haven't been that many Caucasian women giving birth lately . . ."

And seeing my bewildered look: "The Ethiopian women usually organize theirs at church. And the Vietnamese and Chinese women have their own support systems in place."

These closed systems segregate us into small parcels— mothers and babies coping with fundamentally similar circumstances in sometimes radically different ways. I wonder about these other mothers as I see them walking toward me in the park, most often with their babies covered by screens or light blankets draped over the front of their prams. The Vietnamese mothers in particular seem paranoid about the sun, barely letting it fall on their babies' skin. I get told off by an old man outside the market for taking Owen for a five-minute walk to the pharmacy in full view of the sky.

Are these women like me, are they swiftly sinking, too? I do not ask and I do not have the language to ask; in my plummeting state I cannot seem to get my voice to reach beyond the surface of my skin.

When I later try to figure it out, there is no clear answer to be found. Cross-cultural studies on the subject are only just coming into being, qualitative research admitted into the study of women's experiences after years of being considered "fringe." Anthropological findings from the early '80s seemed to determine that postpartum mental illness is a Western issue only; that the postpartum rituals of other countries, built around succoring and honoring the mother and newborn child, successfully inured them from disease. But more recent studies suggest that these results came from the fact that non-Western women don't often *conceptualize* postpartum sadness and fear as being medical rather than cultural.

The EPDS questionnaire I fill in at the maternal and child health nurse's office seems so far to be the best study tool cross-culturally, with its ten weighted questions of behavior and mood:

I have been able to laugh and see the funny side of things:

- As much as I always could
- Not quite as much now
- Definitely not so much now
- Not at all

I have blamed myself unnecessarily when things went wrong; I have felt scared or panicky for no good reason; I have been so unhappy that I have had trouble sleeping.

When the questionnaire is translated into other languages, the responses across study populations are remarkably stable; conservatively, at least one woman in ten scores high enough on this questionnaire to be considered seriously depressed cross-culturally, with the figure rising to about one in seven when self-reporting is conducted in Western nations. I think about all the women I see walking around Footscray, and the women who would have been forcibly removed from this land once, and their descendants, and wonder how they are coping and whether there is a language for their suffering.

I read Dana Jack, on the self-silencing behavior that comes with severe depression. To the nexus of selfhood and social pressure, she brings the brunt of feminist thought to bear:

> Self-silencing is prescribed by norms, values, and images dictating what women are "supposed" to be like: pleasing, unselfish, loving. As I listened to the inner dialogues of depressed women, I heard self-monitoring and negative self-evaluation in arguments between the "I" (a voice of the self) and the "Over-Eye" (the cultural, moralistic voice that condemns the self for departing from culturally prescribed "shoulds"). The imperatives of the Over-Eye regarding women's goodness are strengthened by the social reality of women's subordination . . . Inwardly, they experienced anger and confusion while outwardly presenting a pleasing, compliant self trying to live up to cultural standards of a good woman in the midst of fraying relationships, violence, and lives that were falling apart.[6]

In the time that I am sick, nobody tells me that I am a bad mother. Nobody tells me that my history of depression means that I should never have risked having a child, though I overhear friends talking about the fact that they don't want their children inheriting their genes, their own illnesses, and I wonder what it says about me that I took this risk so blithely. In an op-shop, I find a tattered, outdated chapbook, *Best Psychiatric Jokes*, and read a one-liner:

> A neurotic is a man with both feet planted firmly in thin air.

I don't know whether it is impulse or stupidity or love that has put me in this position; whether it is a desire to hurt myself by walking out into nothingness, out over a ledge. Perhaps until the very moment I fall, I do not believe that it will hurt, or hurt enough. I am lucky, if wanting to die is lucky, that my illness is culturally sanctioned by the Over-Eye; it is not just that I am culturally, acceptedly neurotic, but that my face is the face of the suffering women's canon. Virginia Woolf, Sylvia Plath, Winona Ryder in *Girl Interrupted*: the tragic and creative white woman is such a well-known figure that our fragility and need for protection is automatically assumed—I know walking out over a ledge that there will most likely be somebody there to catch me.

I know this isn't the case for everybody, and I know how few resources there are out there. I know that others need this help as much or more, but I have long ago lost the ability to feel shame about my choices. I have my white skin, my eyes that are green from crying, my polished middle-class vocabulary, and my nice home and healthy white child. My whiteness is a tool in my arsenal and I use it for all that it is worth, because it is one of the things that gets me sympathy and attention, and, ultimately, the means to stay alive.

At the same time, I can't stop thinking about these other women, the ones who don't have recourse to benign stereotypes, only harmful ones, who are supposed to be better at suffering, or more accustomed to it, anyway. There are women for whom the Over-Eye is judgmental and pervasive, the result of political, physical, and social marginalization that is very present and very real; women who are rightly wary of doctors, whose families expect their constant strength or whose priests simply ask them for more faith in God. And I wonder how they cope and how their children cope.

When I think of these women, I do not wish to speak for them, or over them. The urge to raise your voice on behalf of others is one of the double-edged swords of learning to be white; as much as women self-silence, other women sometimes take up their space. So I do not wish to speak on behalf of these women, whose communities close ranks around them protectively, who wander by the river with their heads full of clouds or dreams. It is just that the problem goes so far, it spreads so wide. And I feel that at least part of my life's work is to bear witness.

• • •

When I try to unravel what became of my Judaism, I can follow the threads back to adolescence, the time when my parents steer me away from it the most.

"We wanted to keep you away from the poetry of it," my mother says years later, though I can't remember in what context. For what she and my father intend, it is smart. We always have a Christmas tree and a menorah, an Easter and Seder, and they tell us tolerantly that we can choose what we want to be when we grow up. But all along there is the Father Christmas problem. If you grow up believing in God and are never disabused, that is one thing; but how can you choose to believe if He has never been in your heart?

My Jewish psychiatrist nearly falls out of his chair laughing when I ask him about this. "You don't have to believe in God!" he says. "*Of course* you can be a secular Jew."

I am in my late twenties, and it is almost the very first time I have heard the term. With all of my busy analyzing and unpicking and deconstructing, it has still never occurred to me that some of the things I learned before I knew what they *meant* were wrong. It doesn't matter that my father married out, because everybody bar my grandparents' congregation recognizes patrilineal Jews. *Israel* recognizes patrilineal Jews. A belief in God is not anywhere close to mandatory. If I had stopped to think about it, if I had really asked questions about it, I could have saved myself years of feeling as though I didn't really belong.

But I suspect it goes deeper than that. I think of Paulina, insisting to her atheist parents that she be baptized in the Catholic Church, and posing for photos in a puffy white dress. It's sweet and it's funny, but I think her actions were also sensible. I have made it this far in my life without a belief in God, but I am not strong enough for a life without the existence of ritual.

Mostly I long for the consolation of a foundational good act. A bar or bat mitzvah is essentially this—an agreement with the community and God to obey law, which is knowledge, and to be responsible for your actions; to perform mitzvoth—good deeds—in order to enrich the community and prepare the world for a more holy day. It is also your responsibility to atone, on Yom Kippur; without a dedicated day of atonement I find I get wrapped up in grieving, with a sense of furious helplessness, the things my white skin and good education and enough money represent.

There is no such thing as "good enough," I suspect, because "good enough" is a state of grace. I don't know if I will ever stop feeling as though I am a double agent. That is the privilege of passing; it makes you invisible. In Australia, far from the rest of the world, it can feel like an academic argument, but I look at the rise of anti-Semitism in Hungary and in Poland, and the voters who rally behind American presidential candidates with white supremacist slogans and tattoos,[7] and know that I might not be able to hide in plain sight forever. And I wonder whether the fact that I can and that I do makes me cowardly, or craven, or just pragmatic, and tired of arguing.

Today is Rosh Hashanah, and I think of my grandfather, lightly, as I walk through the blossoming backstreets. Rosh Hashanah, the New Year, marks the day Papa died, after a long slow week in which we all gathered around him. Today, front yards are overflowing with bloom, little buds trusting that the thin warmth of early September sunshine will strengthen and nourish their transition into flowers.

I have trouble remembering the actual date of Papa's death; the Jewish holidays float, they are not stable signifiers. I try to learn the turn of the year by the natural world. Here in Kulin country, Melbourne, the year hinges on the turn of the seven seasons, and the two overlapping seasons of flood and fire. *Iuk* (eel); *Waring* (wombat); *Guling* (orchid); *Poorneet* (tadpole); *Buath Gurru* (grass-flowering season); kangaroo apple; *Biderap* (dry season).[8] There are life cycles that are closely observed, times of scarcity and of abundance. It seems infinitely more sensible than our imported calendar year, with its public holidays for Christmas and Easter, horse races and football matches.

The law says that any branch overhanging a boundary is a common good; it is the rule of summer harvests in the inner suburbs. For years, Mike thought that I was brazenly stealing lemons and pomegranates from our neighbors, not understanding how the system worked. Now I gather armfuls of the natives that have presaged the blossoms in their confidence. I take a sprig here, a sprig there. By the time I arrive home, my arms are overflowing with wax and prickly wattle.

Before my grandparents bought their house, its land had been part of a large, sprawling orchard. Deep root systems connected the earth between their backyard and the neighboring yeshiva. The plants of my childhood memory there were utilitarian; a lemon tree big enough to nestle in, two vast swaths of ivy covering the bookends of a clothesline. Now my mother is making over the garden in rambling color, overwriting its history, once again, with olive trees, a fig, kitchen herbs, and a jacaranda.

Those growths and overgrowths are a wind blowing a few fragments of sand across the surface of a rock, nothing more. In the long view of history, I know that I am an ant, and this thought is oddly comforting. But of course it's just a theory that time travels in one direction, or "travels" at all. It's funny how linked the language of the passage of time is with the idea of heading elsewhere, journeying, meandering—how shot through with the logics of motion.

I find, too, that to write about walking is to come across all kinds of metaphors involving feet and shoes. A lot of them are to do with independence: *to pull oneself up by one's bootstraps*, for example, or *to stand on your own two feet*. Others have to do with empathy: to *put yourself in someone else's shoes*, or *walk a mile* in them. But the one I keep coming back to embodies the ambiguity and ambivalence of my own position, with its undertones of split allegiance. It is that I have *a foot in both camps*.

When I open my computer after getting home, I find an op-ed an American rabbi, Gil Steinlauf, has written for *The Washington Post*, adapted from his Rosh Hashanah sermon. In it, he calls on Jews to abandon their whiteness, having gained everything from it, in order to be representative of a God invested in equality and tolerance. I am struck not just by the extreme clarity of the message, but by his positioning of the feeling of living in an existential border territory as being innate to the work of being a Jew:

> Through the centuries, our moments of power have been all too fleeting. Mostly, our hope has been to be tolerated. From our place at the periphery, we have responded always with the ability to critique injustice, to adopt the cause of the oppressed, to envision a better and more just world. Even in times when we participated fully in non-Jewish societies, we always knew that we stood with one foot in the mainstream, and one foot outside.[9]

It is idealistic, but it is the kind of idealism I clutch on to, in order to keep myself and my treacherous body in check. As I get older, I think sometimes about finding a Progressive congregation, perhaps with a radical feminist rabbi, someone to talk to about this feeling of always encompassing division of some kind. I want my son to grow up feeling Jewish, whatever that is; but not the unwavering Orthodoxy of my grandfather, nor Dad's symmetrical intolerance of its excesses.

I want Owen to grow up with a sense of being something other than male and white, not just for political reasons but because there *is* something else, innate to me, that I still struggle to express. I want him to sit at a Seder table waiting nervously to stumble his Hebrew and ask the four questions, and to learn that our bread is flat because, fleeing as slaves, there was no time for it to rise; that we eat bitter herbs to remind us of the bitterness of slavery; that we dip our food in salt water, then honey, to symbolize the replacement of our tears with gratitude for the sweetness of our freedom; that we recline on our cushions because we can do so—we are free.

Because Dad is so contrary, he has named himself as a grandfather not Papa, but Opa. "A German name!" says my grandmother in disgust. "It's what Greeks say as they smash their plates," he tells her in response. Occasionally we still take walks together, him pushing Owen along briskly to set the pace. Our conversations are more mellow now that I have a child, and now that he has seen me go to a place of sheer helplessness, where I am not equipped with stinging barbs or witty replies. There are still small barbs— things don't change entirely—but they are little barbs of love that bind me to his side.

On the days I work, I take Owen to my parents' place,

and he and my mum romp and play, and often visit Nagyi in her small flat. After her own fall, she moved out of the house, which my parents are renovating so that she can return when the day comes, with a chair to take her up and down the stairs. Owen learns to walk more or less in the corridors of Sheridan Hall, leaning on Nagyi's Zimmer frame for support as he stumbles over his feet.

Mum sends me proof-of-life photos during the day. When Dad gets home he sits in his customary place on the couch, and Owen wiggles up beside him. From time to time I receive a photo of them sitting side by side, Dad eating his almonds and reading the paper, Owen "reading" a book of his own. In the background, I know, at a low hum, the footy is on. Owen snuggles into Dad, into the softness of one of his old, ratty jumpers, and I know exactly what scent he will be breathing in, as I know the scent of my son's milky head. It is the same jumper Dad used to wear in the mornings at least twenty-five years ago. It is more or less disintegrating into threads now, but no one can convince him to throw it out.

RINGS

KNOW THAT it is love because I haven't gone looking for Mike, nor would I have known him if I'd found him. The ex-boyfriend of a friend of mine—she was the barista at the café where I waitressed—he does not occupy a large role in my life. I have served him sausage rolls, watched him waiting patiently outside as Tilly and I did the close, once or twice chatted with him over dinner at their house. He is just a figure, so when he emails, out of the blue, having returned from his peacekeeping mission and from traveling the world, I do not suspect it will be love. How can I? I am twenty-one years old.

I have been in love before, and had my heart ground to shards. I have been ill on and off this year, and I am desperately lonely; it is a dangerous time for my heart, and so I have protected myself, giving in to the occasional fling, but nothing that has had the potential to hurt. Mike seems safe, and I know already that he's kind. He has a "spare ticket" to see David Sedaris; he has remembered how much I love books. I spend the afternoon reading short stories at my friend Zoe's house, narrowing down the short list for a prize.

Mike is evasive over email, keeping the conversation light—for fear, he tells me later, that I might turn him down.

"So, is it a date?" Zoe asks, red pen skittering over the page.

"I have absolutely no fucking clue."

We are supposed to meet at eight, but he turns up at six, finding me where I'd told him I would be, at a friend's poetry gig. Josephine stands on the stage, her clear voice ringing out, and Mike sits by my side. I can feel his attention half on me and half on her; he has never been to a spoken word show before, but his face is open, intent, and when he moves to applaud it is spontaneous and real. When he leaves briefly to get us both a drink, Zoe raises her eyebrow and gives me a tiny nod.

It is funny—I cannot say whether he is attractive or not. I like his clear blue eyes, the breadth of his shoulders. His face is a trick face, all angles, with a scar that bites through his lower lip and a crooked smile that is quick and ready. Studying his sleeping face in the moonlight later, I notice a few lashes missing from his left eyelid, which leave a funny naked dent in the shadow on his cheekbone.

I meet with Josephine a few days later for breakfast.

"I just don't know if I'm ready to get into something big," I say.

She puts down her coffee, giving me an appraising look.

"Jessica, don't put the cart before the horse."

But I know; and he does as well. Standing under a streetlight, waiting to hail a cab, I feel as though all the blood in my body is rushing out toward him. I look at him, and he looks at me, and, almost imperceptibly, things are settled. When we sleep together, the sex feels like a precursor to waking in his arms, where I feel more secure than I have any right to be. Eighteen months later we are married.

I have never thought that I would bother with marriage; if I have any hazily defined plans, they involve wafting around Paris or Berlin, writing a novel, having affairs with older men, or possibly loving someone, moving in with them, having a child together; marriage hasn't seemed necessary. Even now I cannot articulate why I want it. I want it even though I know, intellectually, that a marriage certificate is simply a piece of paper. I know the history of the institution, how oppressive it has been to women, how oppressive it is now to my queer friends who want, if not the institution itself, then at least the right to participate in it. But these things pale before an urge that comes from nowhere, and is as relentless and compelling as the urge to have a baby soon will be.

What I don't want is a wedding. It is a mark of how much Mike loves me that he readily accepts this. He is more community-minded than I am, more generous—it does not make him shrivel to imagine the scrutiny of our families and closest friends, watching with intense love and pride as we exchange words that are private and binding, a compact only for us. I have been having panic attacks daily for weeks now, and he knows how much I fear being the center of attention, any attention.

Instead, we go to the registry, telling our friends and family only afterward. My father, with three daughters, is feminist enough to have been irked by the joking comments of his friends while we were growing—"Better start saving for the weddings now!" He joked throughout our childhoods that if we ever wanted to get married, he would give us a ladder and a check. Upon hearing the news he laughs, and opens a bottle of sparkling wine; the joke is on him, a little, but he has seen how glowingly happy I am, and he likes Mike. "He's like an island of sanity in the ocean of your life," he says. I feel this, too.

I know that Mike is the man for me, in part because he is a sensitive man. Anaïs Nin's essay "In Favor of the Sensitive Man" is a touchstone, one I come back to again and again. Written for *Playgirl* in 1974, it is a treatise on the New Woman—independent, sexually liberated, and liberated by psychotherapy—and her shifting relationships with her male lovers. The Sensitive Man, crucially, disdains the harmful and violent strains of the patriarchy, embracing instead the "feminine" qualities of compassion, communication, and collaborative decision making. Nin describes the relationships she comes across on college campuses:

> They helped each other through college, they answered each other's poems, they wrote confessional and self-examining letters, they prized their relationship, they gave care to it, time, attention. They did not like impersonal sensuality. Both wanted to work at something they loved.
>
> I met many couples who fitted this description. Neither one dominated. Each one worked at what he did best, shared labors, unobtrusively, without need to establish roles or boundaries. The characteristic trait was gentleness. There was no head of the house. There was no need to assert which one was the supplier of income. They had learned the subtle art of oscillation, which is human. Neither strength nor weakness is a fixed quality. We all have our days of strength and weakness. They had learned rhythm, suppleness, relativity.[1]

I love the clarity of this description, the emphasis on a relationship encompassing qualities that shift between its bearers as each can carry them. This is how we begin, and without a child it is easy—mostly. But two fault lines run through our marriage that, if left unattended, could crack it wide apart.

The first is simple, ordinary: "Both wanted to work at something they loved." When we meet, I am young, but my feet are already on the path. I have edited the student paper, I have launched out with Gillian and Caroline on our own journal; the week before my first date with Mike, I enter my first poetry slam, the Doris Leadbetter Poetry Cup, and win. It is clear to me that language is more than a comfort; it will be a life. Mike encourages me to enroll in an honors thesis when the time comes, and I grapple with critical theory, and read and delve in the morning when he goes out to teach, sitting at our dining table, which doubles as my study. I clear the table before he gets home, and get dinner on the stove. Our run-down apartment is full of books and flowers.

Next door, Josephine works at her exquisite short stories. She claimed the apartment for us when it came up for lease, and slowly works on moving her friends in when other apartments come up: Chris and Eirian; Gra; for a short time, Lorelei. Chris and Lorelei are writers, too, Eirian, a graphic designer, and the second floor of our building is a constant whir of books passed back and forth, dinner parties, coffee, fortnightly trips to the pub down the road where Josephine and Chris run a storytelling night. Mike plays guitar, and noodles around, writing songs. His work is merely a day job. He doesn't grudge my not earning an income, but he is the odd man out here and it chews away at him, this lack of an anchoring craft.

The building is sold out from under us, and we spread out across the city, newly atomized. I finish my thesis and look for a job, waiting for my results to come back. When they do come they are so good that I write to my supervisor asking if there has been a mistake. There hasn't. Mike comes to the award ceremony, and is impressed by the quality of the canapés.

The idea of him returning to study has been floating around for a while now, but it begins to solidify. For a while he thinks he might like to study law, but he flunks the LSAT, not understanding that people study for it for years; that it is not simply a test of raw aptitude, but an industry in and of itself. His focus shifts, and he scrapes into a master's in international relations by the skin of his teeth. Most of his BA was spent writing plays, bartending, and falling in love; his marks are not exceptional. But the application goes well; he is buoyed up by his sturdiness, his quickness of response. He knuckles down to study, and I go out to work, juggling jobs at two different journals, and I hope against hope that his restlessness will be stilled.

After the elopement, our parents insist on throwing us a party, one in which we will celebrate with our community and allow them to give us gifts, against which I had initially demurred. It is lovely, held on a sunny winter afternoon in my parents' back garden. I am running on high tension all day—my hair is wrong, my face is wrong, my cheeks hurt from smiling—but I keep a lid on it, drawing from the warming glow of people's obvious delight for us. When the anxiety hits and it gets too hard to manage, I lock myself in the bathroom, breathe deeply, splash water on my face, and emerge for a glass of champagne. The alcohol helps; it depresses the nerves, and it's better to be a tipsy bride than a distraught one.

My little sisters stand on a garden bench and make a speech, which brings me to tears. Mike cries on and off all day, but then he is a soft touch, Irish sentimentality rooted deep within him. Claire and Olivia take it in turns to speak, passing a piece of A4 printer paper between them. Olivia starts:

> After eighteen and twenty-one years respectively
> of knowing Jess, we thought we had her pegged;
> so when she told us she was bringing over her
> new boyfriend, Mike—a blue-eyed, Californian
> bartender from the army—it's fair to say we were
> thrown . . .

Mike joined the Army Reserve at seventeen, newly arrived back from a nine-year stint in the United States. It's something that I've never really understood, and so I've pushed it to the back of my mind, where it will not trouble me. I know it is connected with service, with a feeling of needing to contribute something, but the military is so far from my daily life of books and art and criticism that I prefer not to think about it. Every Tuesday night Mike disappears for Parade, and I am reminded each time that there is a side of him that I cannot connect to, from which I am shut out.

This is the second fracture line: the hairline crack in the way we approach our ethics that unsettles and unnerves me when I look at it under glass. For me, patriotism has always expressed itself as critique, a pushing back against successive governments that are taking the country inexorably toward neoliberalism, at the expense of social welfare and human rights. I find Mike's willingness to throw himself into a hierarchy troubling; there is no room for dissent there. I do not want him to be absorbed into "something bigger." When somebody tells him to jump, I do not want him to ask how high.

Halfway through the master's I find out I am pregnant. I am overjoyed. At this point I am only planning to take leave from my job, not to leave it completely; Mike will continue to study part-time and maybe teach a little, so that he can spend time at home with the baby. It is in keeping with our spirit of egalitarianism—neither one of us wants me to default to being a stay-at-home mother, me because I am too ambitious and truly love my job, Mike because he doesn't want to miss out on these first few months. He wants the full experience of having a baby. He wants to get up in the night to change it, feed it, rock it to sleep; to take it to its appointments in the day, and walk through the park, and have coffee down the road with a sleeping child strapped to his chest.

The weeks pass, and Mike throws himself into study. He has found an unlikely passion—the politics of international space asset cooperation, and the effects of terrestrial competition and collaboration on the ability of nations to preserve the security of their space technologies. He subscribes to *Aviation Week and Space Technology*. It astounds me that there is enough news in this area for a weekly periodical.

I come from a family of girls; I am one of three, my mother is one of three. I feel sure that this baby blossoming beneath my skin will be a little girl. Mike comes from a family of boys; he is one of two, his father one of four. As the baby grows, we joke about whose DNA will be prevalent. If it is a girl, I plan to name her Coralie, after my bohemian auntie Coralie, really a great-great-aunt, whose deco bangles and marriage-that-wasn't-a-marriage thrilled me as a child.

It's a boy. At twenty weeks, the sonographer is able to tell by a glance, even though she has been careful to angle the scope so that we cannot see genitalia unless we want to. A boy! My stomach drops. I can't fathom my dismay—it comes from deep inside me, from somewhere other than the space in which my baby resides. I am confident I can raise a kind, fierce, feminist daughter; I know firsthand the things against which to guard her. But my experience of men is only from the outside, and the phrase that keeps ringing in my head is *toxic masculinity*.

I think about footy clubs and locker rooms, about men

punching each other on the arm jovially, and telling each other, "Harden up, princess." I think about gang rape and blurred lines and barbecues and beer and the army, and calling each other Steve-o and Jonesy, and all the little jokes about women that are not really jokes at all; I think about little girls being told that if a boy pulls their hair he must like her; about the dwindling number of boys in my ballet class, and the torturous schoolyards of my queer male friends.

Mike takes me by the hand and tries to calm me down.

"Darling, it will be okay. We'll raise him to be a good man. I played footy as a child and I'm *fine*."

And he is, I know. He is funny and caring and sweet; and every Tuesday night he marches in formation, with a gun.

Owen arrives, and Mike's workload doubles, more than doubles. He has taken on a minor thesis within his course work, so as to keep the pathway to a PhD open, which I am quietly thrilled about. I build us a fantasy future in the inner suburbs, Mike cycling to the university every day to teach, me working on the staff of a prestigious magazine. Mike is a good teacher, an excellent one even, but teaching is not his passion—research is. He throws himself into his thesis and spends more and more time at the library. At the same time, I begin to sink.

Alone at home with the baby, my days lose their sense

of proportion. I tell myself that what I have is good, better than if Mike was working a nine-to-five; he is there in the middle of the night, he changes nappies, he sings to Owen and genuinely adores him. But he cannot be there every minute, and the minutes are beginning to expand. Soon, as well as taking care of Owen, he is taking care of me.

I resent bitterly the time he spends away from us. Mike tells me with enthusiasm about the essays he is writing, and I have to grit my teeth to keep from biting out some nasty comment about the amount of time it takes him to finish them. I remember how little I discussed my own thesis with him, how outcast he felt at the time from the language of scholarship and theory, and how carefully I kept my excitement to myself; but he is absorbed now, enthused, and more important, neither of us has anything else to discuss except the baby, and we are both immersed in the baby—there is little to be said that we have not already shared.

Eventually the thesis is done, handed in. Now it is his turn to job hunt. There are graduate programs in Melbourne, but they are not the exciting ones. His friends are flying up for interviews in Canberra. He sends out application after application, but his late return to academia is against him, and with a baby at home he has had no time for the extras: volunteering, unpaid internships. This is a field in which every moment counts.

A few weeks later he sits at the table, refreshing the screen on the laptop until his results come back. I take a glance and let out a whoop.

"Mazel tov!" I yell, bending over to cradle his head in a hug. "You must be so excited!"

"Yeah," he says slowly, "it's a good mark." He looks at me blankly, trying to raise a grin. "I mean, not as good as *yours* . . . but . . ."

And even though he means it as a joke, it goes right through my flesh and he knows it. All this time, we have gone back and forth—it is the same argument over and over again.

"You don't understand—you *have* a career! You know what it's like to be successful at something you love. I've never had that."

"*You* don't know what you're asking me to give up!"

I try to keep the hurt off my face, knowing this is shaky ground. I cannot listen to him denigrate this accomplishment, denigrate me; for what have I picked up the slack at home while he studied if this degree means nothing to him, cannot satisfy him? I have hoped that the master's would fill whatever gap there was that could only be plugged by work, but it has just become evident we cannot both have work we dearly love, at least not at the same time.

A military job will give Mike the stability he craves, the sense of making a difference. But it will make me a helpmeet, a wife. I will go to formal dinners and I will arrange house moves, and I will be picked up and put down in different states when his work requires it. Training will take him away from me and from Owen; I will have to be a full-time carer in those weeks and months, or work to be able to afford the day care I will need in order to work. I can freelance, but I will not be able to commit to a magazine job, not without knowing where I will be living the next year. There are few bases in Melbourne; we will likely have to move.

Later that night he comes to lie beside me, holding my face very gently with our noses almost touching.

"I know how much I am asking you to give up," he says. "That's how I know this is real. I would never put you through this if I didn't *need* to."

And my castles in the air capitulate in the face of his desperation. I cannot give him much, broken and exhausted as I am, but I can give him the means to assuage his plummeting self-respect.

He leaves on a hot day in January, out of contact for at least a fortnight, limited to a brief conversation every evening after that. For the next three months, it is Owen and it is me. Our lives become smaller in the absence of a second parent; we are shrunk down to a unit of two.

Every morning, when Owen wakes up, he climbs out of his bed and comes to get me, his little weight hanging off the door handle as he swings his way into the room. From there, there is a ritual: take a sip of my water; put my glasses on my still half-sleeping face; play with my wedding rings, sitting one on top of the other next to the bed, and then push them determinedly onto my finger.

Inside the house, this finger is often naked. Doing the

dishes, or taking a shower, or typing, means rings left haphazardly on window ledges or next to the computer, all the
better for small fingers to find. Outside, without them, I
feel exposed, the bare skin on my left ring finger heavier
and more raw to the elements than it should be. My hand
is out of kilter, it has the wrong weight, and the off-balance
between left and right throws my whole body out of sorts.

In the off-hours, hauling a toddler around or loading
laundry into the machine, I savor lines of the intermittent
emails Mike is able to send.

> There is so much that I want to tell you. Every
> day some absurd thing happens and everyone
> here treats it as normal and my first instinct is to
> tell you about it, but by the time I get to a
> computer or my phone three or four different
> absurd things have happened and pushed it out of
> my memory. Give Owen a hug and a kiss for me.

And

> There was a rumor the other day that the
> military working dogs were out exercising, and
> it made me think of our future happy dog, and
> backyard, and going for walks along a leafy
> suburban street early in the morning. I think
> about Owen playing with his first dog. I think
> about you and Owen. I think about how big he's
> getting, and the way that you look when you're

asleep. I think about what it was like to be at the park around the corner on warm spring afternoons, and cooking for you, and riding down to Blackhearts with Owen on the bike to buy a bottle of wine for a dinner party.

And

I love you I love you I love you.
And my hair is growing back.

But our phone calls are infrequent, and the sense of his absence grows. I try to find the comfort in these phone calls, which we make at six p.m. so that Mike can hear Owen's voice. "Daddy!" he exclaims, then goes back to playing with his plastic tow truck. At two and a half he is still young enough to believe that Daddy lives in the phone sometimes. Sometimes he lives in the iPad, where Mike appears on-screen, reading stories we recorded a few weeks back. A Daddy is omnipresent, existing in all states.

A husband, though, needs to be physically present; where I go to draw comfort from the fact of loving him, there is nothing but air. I miss the bulk of his body walking through the door, breaking the circuits of tension that have grown between Owen and me during the day. Owen is possessive, I am desperate for five minutes alone— I need to regain a sense of my own physical autonomy, the limits of my body, which Owen confuses or presumes for his own. It is perverse, but I need somebody else to grant me the permission of solitude.

At night Owen grabs my hands and plumps them under his cheeks. I have become a living pillow, a blanket, and it is profoundly beautiful and sweet; I know how precious is the trust I have been given. But at the same time, my days are lacking in balance, growing perilously small.

One afternoon I get an email I've been hoping for: after three consecutive applications, I've finally been successful with a writing grant. Relief floods through me at the prospect of paying off our debt, of not having to find shift work while Mike is still away; of being able to *work*, to send Owen to day care and cover the cost, to get a haircut and finally fix the track pad on my computer. I text Mike, and grab a bottle of wine on the way home. Later that night, Owen poos in the bath.

I cannot handle shit. I *hate* it. Changing nappies is, by far, the materially worst part of parenthood for me; Mike doesn't mind and does it with aplomb. I wish I had his equanimity. I am missing whatever makes people find scatological humor funny—the Adam Sandler gene. Because there is no one else to do it I attend to Owen's nappies, holding my revulsion in.

"Okay," says Mike when Owen switches to solids from the breast. "You deal with vomit, I'll deal with poo."

But it is no longer either/or. One long hot day Owen

is fractious, in the kind of temper I can't soothe, whimpering and whinging by turns. I take him for a long walk, hoping to lull him to sleep, and as my shins are beginning to ache, he quiets—and then the sookiness starts up again, amping up into an outraged wail. Just as we reach home he arches his back and spews down the side of the pusher, all over himself.

"Oh, darling," I say as my heart sinks. "It's okay. Mummy's here. You're okay!"

I scoop him up and bundle off his T-shirt, trying to keep the vomit out of his hair. I cross my fingers as I carry him up two flights of stairs, praying that none of our neighbors will come home and have to pick through his vomit to get to the entryway. Owen has barely touched food all day, but bottles of milk have curdled into soupy white chunks that dot the footpath right outside the door.

I put him in the bath, soothe him, wipe him down with a face washer, then tuck him into bed, a laptop set up on a chair halfway across the room. When he curls up, exhausted, and *Play School* has his attention, I race down the stairs with a saucepan full of cool soapy water, cursing the fact that there are no taps outside. Dragging the pusher into the patch of dirt that passes for a garden I sluice it down, then race upstairs again; check that Owen is okay, race down, sluice, getting the footpath as clean as I possibly can. After twenty minutes Owen is dozing, and I am crouched in the garden, trying to get vomit out of the safety buckle of the pusher with an old toothbrush and a sponge.

Now I pluck Owen from the bath and wrap him in a

towel, imploring him to stay put. He doesn't, of course, but follows me into the kitchen, towel trailing behind him, as I grab an old takeaway container and go fishing around the bath for his decomposing turds. I scoop them up, and he dances with glee as I flush them down the toilet.

"A big poo!" he tells me, face suffused with pleasure at his own cleverness. "A big, big poo!"

You owe me, I tell Mike fiercely in my head, as though somehow he could have spared me this: the ordinary work of being a mother. When Owen has gone to sleep, I drink the whole bottle of wine.

My mother takes Owen for a few days so I can fly up for Mike's graduation ceremony, an expense the air force meets. On the plane, I watch the sun bounce off the facets of the diamonds in my ring, making small galaxies of light jump when I move my hand. Three black diamonds in a band of thin white gold; Mike bought the ring for me online, at a police auction in the States, and his father forwarded it to our little house in St. Kilda. I didn't think about an engagement ring, since we skipped the engagement completely, but I had bought Mike a wedding band, and he wanted to give me something in return.

My own wedding band I made myself, when I was eleven years old, softening a strip of sterling silver over a Bunsen burner and then polishing it up as a Christmas present for my mother. She returned it to me much later when we came across it cleaning out the house—her rings are family rings, and made of gold—and this is the ring that Mike took off my finger and put back on again, as the smell of sulfur from exploded fireworks mingled with the smell of flowers, in the gardens in Jolimont where we saw in our first New Year together.

We had made the decision together that morning, quietly, sitting across the table from each other at Mike's favorite café. *What do you want to do with the New Year? I think we should get married.* It would be another thirteen months before we could scrape together the registry fee. In the gardens, as he "proposed" through a whirl of champagne and light and hilarity, he did so knowing full well that we had made the choice together.

Three days prior to the flight, Owen makes off with both rings, and I go nearly frantic trying to find them. After two anxious nights I find them hidden in a slit in the couch, not just beneath the cushions but buried deep in the solid mass of wood and springs and leather. I take a photo and send it to Mike, telegraphing my relief. On the plane to go and meet him, I look at my hand, and I cannot tell if it's the movement of the plane or if I, myself, am trembling.

It has started to drizzle by the time I get to the base the next day. I keep my taxi receipt to be reimbursed and make my way to the grandstand, feeling already too brittle for the noise, the color, the mass of people congregated in the midst of a vast expanse of concrete and dry grass. Behind me a small family jokes and feeds chocolate biscuits to a toddler, trying to keep him from going exploring beneath the bleachers, and I am stabbed by longing for my impossible, unruly child.

A brass band comes on, marching all in air force blue, playing "The Girl from Ipanema." Then two clusters of stiff figures, marching in formation, legs the same, stiff backs the same, faces shaved; from a distance the women's faces are interchangeable with the men's. All around me people cheer and wave; one couple sits transfixed, watching the procession through a video camera, and I fight back tears as I look for Mike's loping shoulders-forward walk, now stifled, his beard now gone; I look and look, but I cannot pick out his face from the rows of faraway faces. In these lines of marching blue he is nowhere.

After the ceremony is over, a voice through a megaphone tells us where lunch will be served; we move off, in dribs and drabs, as the blue figures recede. I have walked to the parade ground down a strip called Values Avenue, and follow it up again now. The values, printed on flags that whip in the wind, are: Respect, Excellence, Agility, Dedication, Integrity, and Teamwork.

Beyond the flags, a conference room is lined in sandwich trays; loud figures laugh and chatter and eat party pies out of heated basins, heedless of the fact that our sons and husbands and daughters aren't with us yet. A man in pristine sailors' whites carries around an oversized pink lamington. I ask a figure in blue when we will see them, our loved ones; ten minutes, he reckons.

Ten minutes grows to fifteen, and then to forty. I walk

into the women's bathroom and stand in a cubicle, trying to feel my feet inside my shoes, my skin barely keeping the boundaries of my body together. I bite the inside of my cheek down hard, trying to channel my panic into the pain, but the pressure is too pervasive, and I feel too hot for my clothes. Outside it is cooler, and I find a hedge where I can stand and pretend to be invisible, my green top and cream headscarf, Virginia's scarf, the colors of the scrub.

When Mike finally finds me, I am standing there, paralyzed. He opens his arms to me, and the tears I have been holding in flood out and I gasp like a little fish, shaking, trying not to smear his service dress with lipstick and tears, horribly aware of the grandmothers and uncles who are averting their eyes, or worse, giving Mike compassionate looks.

"Look," says Mike. "There's another part of the ceremony, but I don't think you should come to it."

"But—I came all this way."

"They're just going to give us a certificate. You should take a taxi home and have a bath."

"I don't think I can have a bath. I think I need a nap."

"I'll come as soon as I can get away."

"Are you sure?"

"Yep."

In the cab back home the driver doesn't talk, and away from the base, the tension releases, and with it I am flooded with a deep, deep sense of having failed; having failed to keep it together, even for one afternoon. Even more deeply, I feel the failure of not *wanting* this for Mike, of loathing the conformity and artifice and mindless obedience the ceremony has seemed to represent, and feeling it beneath him. I know that that feeling only reflects on my snobbery, but I am unable to see past it.

By the time I get back to the cottage I have rented, I am exhausted by shame. Groggy with sleep already, I get into bed fully clothed. When I wake, it is to Mike gently molding himself to my body, his arm thrown over my waist; he is back in his real clothes, jeans and a checked shirt, and at the feel of his breath against the bare skin of my neck all my love for him floods back, and I am home.

Mike's brother Andrew got married a few months ago, in the Japanese garden of the zoo. Mike got permission to fly down from a new training course—another ten weeks away from home—and his father and stepmother came over from LA. My parents came as well, having grown close to Andrew over the years.

The day was a typical Melbourne day, gray and rainy in the morning, and then obligingly clearing half an hour before the ceremony itself. We could hear loudspeakers announcing the seal-feeding times as Emily, Andrew's fiancée, took her small slow steps down the aisle. I looked at her, hastily turning away from Andrew, whose face was alight with pride and happiness and a faint disbelief.

Mike stood next to him, lean and tanned. Weeks of running and swimming had slimmed him, broadened his shoulders; his eyes were swimming-pool blue against the outdoor brown and pink of his face. I caught his eye as Emily joined the bridal party, and he very slightly winked, turning his attention back to Andrew, prodding him where his brother needed prodding. Andrew, who has Asperger's, had fretted for weeks over getting any part of the ceremony wrong; Mike held the rings and nudged him a few times with his foot, and then tackled him from behind in a bear hug when the music played and the bridesmaids blew streams of bubbles through the air.

Later that night Emily's mother chivied us onto the dance floor, and together we whirled around the bride and groom, in the midst of dancing fathers, mothers, stepparents, cousins, and friends. I looked at Mike's sloping cheeks and crooked mouth and could not imagine ever loving anyone else.

I still worry about how we will balance our life, knowing the raft of factors that are against me. It is easy to speak of taking turns, as we have done, when there is an even playing field; our current plan is that once Owen has finished primary school, Mike will step sideways into a nonprofit or do his PhD, and we will move anywhere in the world I can land a magazine job: Toronto or New York or Berlin. I know, deep down, that this is a fantasy only, no matter our good intentions.

If our life follows the cultural patterns laid out for us—and there is no reason to believe that it won't—Mike will inevitably be promoted during the time I stay at home; the disparity between our hypothetical salaries will grow, which will make it more sensible for him to continue to work, and, if we are not very careful, we will gradually and imperceptibly begin to privilege his career over mine. I will be considered a liability in the workplace for being a mother, whereas Mike will be praised for his devotion to his family, despite the fact that we parent the same child. I will lose touch with the intimate goings-on of my industry, which is hemorrhaging jobs, and bleeding money that the Defense Force will always find in droves.

But these are the broad strokes. Mike holds me as we dance, and I think about all the times I have gone away from him, sunk into anxiety and depression, at times almost catatonic, at others shaking with a rage that wells up out of nowhere and scares him shitless. There are no set times or schedules for when I go away, and he bears the uncertainty with so much grace I cannot understand it, nor the fact that with all things being equal, he would marry me again.

There is, too, a part of him that I will never understand: disciplined, unbending, but ready to bow to somebody else's authority if he thinks it will serve a greater good. There are claims on him that I can no longer afford to be cynical about, knowing how deep within him the need to contribute something to his community runs. And I think of how, having cared for me and for Owen so tenderly, he has left us only temporarily; to make his own way, to give, to be able to provide for a wife who sometimes cannot provide for herself no matter what her politics impel.

I want the first turn because I am terrified that if I do

not take it, there may never be a turn for me again. But I know there *is* a way, and I know it because of this man, this tall, loving man with his regulation haircut and loving, gentle hands. I was right to jump in with both feet; I never had any doubts about the man himself. It is knowing which things to sacrifice, and which things to fight tooth and nail for, that will be the long work of our marriage.

When I try to look into the future the only things I can see are the small ones, seemingly incidental: my hands unpacking boxes and hanging paintings; Mike sweeping pen across paper; Owen's solemn face as he cracks an egg into a bowl. I look at Mike's sleeping body when I wake, and marvel at the ongoingness of his presence in our bed, this solid, freckled pillar of strong bone and love. For the moment, in the richness of a morning, it is vividly, intensely enough.

AINSLIE

WE **ARRIVED IN** Canberra in late December, driving up the Hume with our luggage stacked high in the car. Our furniture had gone ahead of us, put in storage at the air force's expense until we found a suitable house. Owen kicked his legs against the back of my seat, but the kicks meant he wasn't trying to escape his car seat, so I put up with the rhythm of it, the blows muffled by padding as they traveled along my spine.

Staying the night in Yackandandah, I let myself pretend it was a holiday. We had booked a little storybook cottage and exclaimed over it; we cooked pasta on the small stove and sat on the veranda, well sprayed with Rid, beating the old armchairs down first with a broom to get rid of spiders. I curled up with the battered paperback copy of *The Prime of Miss Jean Brodie* I'd bought in an op-shop along the way, trying not to think of the morning's partings, or the city I had left behind.

Leaving the next morning, we slowed, and then swerved, to avoid an echidna waddling across the road. As we drove, the countryside flattened out, the roads widened, the colors turned from dense and complex silvery grays to a drab faded yellow. Coming back into radio reception, the murmurs of talkback were interrupted every ten minutes or so with fire-safety information. The air, when we stopped for a break, was peppery, hot, and dry.

Later that evening, settled into our serviced apartment, I stepped out onto the balcony to watch the sun set. The light was almost eerily peach-toned, spotlighting the dips and curves of a fringe of bluish mountains. The hills circled the city, smudging out the horizon, and I tried to understand how we had come to be so far inland. With the windows open back home, I smelled the rich, sour tang of the sea.

For as long as I can remember I have always lived near water—Melbourne is built on waterways: the Maribyrnong, the Yarra, the bay. I have fed the black swans on the lake in the Botanical Gardens, back when you were allowed to, and tied a bit of sausage on the end of a string for the eels. I have sat on the sand in my bathers, eating hot jam doughnuts, when the height of summer spat jellyfish into the shallows and made swimming itself impossible. I have lain on the bathroom floor, cold tiles against my back, and thought so very longingly about drowning myself in the river.

If you hold a shell to your ear you can hear the ocean, which is, in fact, the gushing tide of your own blood. Take the shell away, and your blood is still there. That is how I felt about the river. I shut my eyes and imagined the weedy water-growth tangled in my hair. When I opened them again and saw the inside of my house, the river was still there, an undertow to my existence in what should have been a safe, snug stronghold.

Feeding Owen, cooking dinner, occasionally seeing friends and laughing with them and keeping up a front— all this happened with the river sucking away at my foundations, the way a house is left rotting from beneath after a flood. When I walked into the wet back garden, desperate to feel the ground beneath my feet, I thought of the rain and how it penetrated deep into the soil, sinking down to water tables, flowing down the steep grassy hill toward the banks below.

When I think about it now, there is a dreamlike quality to this time, as though it doesn't really belong to me. Perhaps this is one of the kindnesses of the brain: "phase blindness," the mechanism that lets you close out a too-strong anguish in the same way you cannot, by thinking about it, reconstruct in your body the sensation of physical pain. I do know that my mother drove me to the hospital. I had an appointment, in Emergency, to inspect my still-inflamed uterus, ballooned up with pain months after the birth, to see if a stronger antibiotic was needed. I sat in the passenger seat with my hands between my lap and the seat belt, trying to ease the bite of its necessary restraint.

I remember, too, my sister crooning to the baby, "I love you. Yes, I *love* you!" and the stab of murderous rage I felt toward her for expressing something I myself couldn't feel. How *dare* she? I trembled with the force of it. All the way to Emergency I hung in the balance between that rage, the physical pain, and a mounting pressure at the base of my throat. Waiting for my appointment, the phone rang, and Owen's wail came tinny and loud through the speaker. She couldn't get him to calm down, my sister said. She couldn't get him to feed. My mother hesitated, and then left, a firm glance at the intake nurse before she went to rescue my child.

With my mother gone, I was free to think. What I thought about, in the white clean glare of the waiting room, was the building where I had once taken French. The university was across the road from the hospital; I could leave right now, walk across the room, walk to the right building and up all eleven flights of stairs, a route I took when the elevators were lurching too erratically to feel safe. The room where French was held had windows that opened wide to the sky, and I used to sit with my hand pressed to the inner wall, terrified of somehow falling out. I could walk to the window now, and simply fall.

I wouldn't even need to walk that far. People get hit all the time, darting across the road; I could time it to look like an accident. With the sharp nail of my thumb I pressed crescents into the skin of my left wrist, trying to bring myself back, but no matter how hard I jammed in the nail I could not draw blood. It took a monumental effort to get up, and I stood for a beat while black dots blinked in and out of the edge of my field of vision. Then I walked over to the triage station.

"I think . . ."

My voice was a croak. I tried again, rolling away the boulder from my throat.

"I think I need to be inside the doors."

The nurse looked at me and passed me a tissue. I hadn't even realized that I was crying; I don't know if you could call it crying. It was as though my body simply released its load of grief, and the tears rolled sharp and salty down my face as if they would never stop.

After Mike came and drove me home, he filled the prescription I had been written, an antidepressant that made me feel half awake again—but only half. Slowly I began to come to the surface of my own life.

I started to visit the wetlands again, walking down through the park and along the river to catch the scent of revegetated marshes. Under the old stock bridge was a mosaic I liked to visit. I pushed on until I reached the temple, then stood still, taking in the grandeur and peace of the Heavenly Queen, whose gold outstretched hand caught the afternoon sun. The planning permissions had just snuck in; built on a floodplain, the temple was surrounded by water, not just the river and the marsh, but the low flat lakes of rain that turned the raw earth to mud as well. Out of the water and silt she rose, Heavenly Queen of Mazu, the goddess of the sea.

When the wind bit too hard, I moved on, leaning on the pusher for support, making sure the blanket around Owen's legs was firmly tucked in. Passing the community center, we finally reached the op-shop, my haven, where Owen opened his big round eyes and took in the bright lights, the loud colors, the glorious heterogeneity of things discarded and donated and cleaned and rearranged, ready to be taken for new uses to new homes.

I couldn't face the two-dollar shops that dotted Nicholson Street, identical in their displays of plastic buckets and cheaply made brooms, folding chairs, bamboo steamers. Going into one of these for a packet of nails or a pair of scissors was agony: I started looking at all the plastic bowls and wondering how many plastic bowls existed in Footscray, in Melbourne, on the earth; I saw the factories where people labored, saw the petrol thick and viscous extracted from great gaping holes in the earth; saw enormous ships laden with flimsy goods crossing the oceans, leaving polluted waters to carry toxins through deep, deep currents to krill and coral and weeds. How many plastic buckets were there in the world, how many bowls?

It calmed me immensely to see some of them at the op-shop, given a second chance. All the mismatched sets of china and three-dollar woolen jumpers had the same provenance as the plastic junk, but at one step's remove I could bear them. It was hypnotic to walk through the racks of clothes and try to imagine the bodies that had animated and filled them. Best, though, most calming, were the racks of books.

Here, a jumble of tastes and inclinations met indiscriminately, shelved in unexpected and sometimes desultory ways—I found Ruth Park's *Swords and Crowns and Rings* in Fantasy. I ran my thumb along the books, feeling the softened edges of old paper yielding beneath my touch. *Trash* and *treasure* are verbs, after all; to cherish, or to discard. Everyone who met here could come away with something, standing appraisingly before the shelves and longing to be transported somewhere new. Sometimes the selection was especially good, and I imagined two lovers settling down together, amalgamating their books, carefully weeding out duplicates they knew would never again be needed.

I wondered how many women had been here before me, babies strapped to their chests, running their thumbs over cracked and broken spines. I had barely any money, or at least no income, but with coins dug out from the bottom of my handbag I could usually buy a book. One book, no more, to justify the hours spent pacing the aisles; to add to a growing library of books overflowing the shelves, grouped in batches or stacks, each waiting to be opened, skimmed through, assimilated, cherished—*read*.

When the antidepressants began to work, enough, I found a part-time job, one I believed that I could do with my brain still at half speed. Money was still running down, though, so we said goodbye to our beloved Footscray and moved to a flat in Balaclava. It was pretty, a small white-washed mews, but the stumping was old and in winter the damp rose through the walls, and slugs came in through the floorboards. Owen's room, at least, was insulated by our bookcase, lined with paperbacks shelved two deep. Every Tuesday and Wednesday my parents walked around to pick Owen up before I left for work, bringing a bagel from Glick's to soothe his impending teeth.

For the first time, too, I had day care. My mother, worried at Owen's lack of social interaction, took him to a playgroup housed at our local maternal and child health center. From there she found a form that I could have filled out—a magic passport to the top of the council waiting list, where vulnerable children waited to skip the immense queues.

This is the part of parenthood where self-esteem gives way to expedience. The language used to describe my situation was a formula that skirted just around a suggestion of neglect; it stung to have to itemize the ways in which I failed as a mother, failed to be healthy enough, trustworthy enough, present; I mentally listed the days on which I had lain in bed while Owen counted spare change into an ice-cream tub on the mattress beside me, and realized that I would have to emerge from limbo and into the light at some point.

I think that I believed then that I was as well as I was ever likely to be; that something was better than nothing, and that a life in which I didn't want to die was worth the sadness, the lost time, the stupor in my limbs. Any change

that might take me back to the way I had been—the terror
and the despair—wasn't worth the risk. It was the first time
I had taken medication, and I didn't know what *well* should
really feel like, so I took the sadness in stride and told myself I was cured; but on a form I still looked negligent of
my child, and on the cusp of crisis; I wasn't *well enough*.

The local GP didn't know much about psychiatric prescription, so he referred me to an outpatient clinic. Two
weeks later I had an appointment with a postpartum psychiatric specialist, a man I initially suspected on the grounds
of being a man, but who looked at me appraisingly and cut
the medical side of my problems down to whole cloth. He
looked at my prescription, and he looked at me, and we
both acknowledged that changes had to be made.

Over months he carefully weaned me off the pills I was
taking, keeping me out of the hospital with sedatives, talking, and trust. A pill in the morning was followed by a pill
at night, and a series of consultations with Kristy, the therapist in the room next door. Neither of them discouraged
Owen from sitting on the floor, babbling as I talked or
didn't talk, his keen little fingers pulling apart their caches
of office toys. Both of them had children of their own. The
receptionist unfailingly offered me coffee when I arrived,
and called taxis for me on the days when my body froze,
made rigid from gentle probing or fatigue or grief, and
always rang to make sure I remembered my appointments
a day ahead of time.

The pill at night made me sleep, and for the first time
in years, I really, consistently, slept. It was amazing to me

how hungry my body was for sleep. Slowly, slowly, the fog began to dissipate, and the sensitivity that had pooled in my eyes and ears and fingertips drew inward toward my heart and mind, where it belonged. Light and sound resumed their right proportion. With the aid of medication and self-care, I was learning to forge new neural pathways.

During our first week in Canberra I was alone. Mike went straight to work, leaving me and Owen to swelter together in our serviced apartment, through the incessant heat. I loathed the building we were housed in for its impersonality, and Canberra for abetting its beige furniture and the TV bolted to the wall. It was homesickness, of course, and fear; after telling myself that I was equal to a new city, I began to worry that I'd left too much of myself behind.

Canberra was a planned city, a top-down infrastructure made for politicians and bureaucrats, where Art and Culture took on capital letters and became monolithic. There would be no meandering here, no slow potter around the old growth of terraces and alleyways; there were few secondhand bookshops, and no tiny shop-front galleries in rows of unleased shops. To live here I would have to move with purpose, and know what that purpose was. I kicked myself for leaving my family, my therapist, my friends, and when I was done kicking myself, Mike made me a gin and tonic and we began to look for somewhere to live.

Our furniture came out of storage, our carefully packaged paintings and our heavy stoneware.

"You got a lot of books," said one of the removalists suspiciously. "Are you a teacher or something?"

"A writer," I said apologetically as he loaded up his dolly with more and more boxes. When the removalists had left and the paperwork had been done, I wandered around the new house, getting to know its doors and windows, the windows that opened out horizontally like garage doors. The house, 1950s navy housing, was built of poured concrete slabs, so all of the wiring was in the ceiling. Owen pretended to be a kangaroo, jumping off the floor, trying to catch the down-hanging light cords.

I made his room up first, sticking his scribbly drawings on the wall. Opening up boxes felt like a lucky dip. I felt wave after wave of gladness assail me as I found things that I hadn't known I was missing: paintings, yes, but also our round, pobby vegetable peeler; a particular bowl with a chip in it; the heavy marble bases of two reading lamps, cast-offs from my parents' house. The wedding china, a gift from my father's best friend; the devil's ivy that Helen grew me from a cutting. All these things had traveled with us to houses and houses, arranged each time in new iterations of a home.

Standing at the kitchen sink, washing a plate or waiting for the kettle to boil, I could see birds foraging around the yellow grass for seed. These birds were streaks of color through the sky as they took flight, varieties of rosella and lorikeet that I had never seen before and couldn't identify. Our bird book was in one of the boxes, waiting to be rediscovered.

There were new things, too, to exult over. I loved the deep laundry sink, the feeling of sloshing bedsheets around in it, up to the elbows in suds made by a slug of eucalyptus oil. When the sheets were done I would carry them into the backyard to peg them out on the Hills Hoist, winding it down to my height and taking in the fresh peppery smell of the grass, the blue plums shaken off the tree. Though most of the garden was lawn, I began to learn its perimeters: the plums, some blue and some golden red, and the apricots overhanging our car space from next door's tree; the bamboo planted by a former tenant; the rosebush whose thorns bit my wrist when I reached into the letter box. I padded out to hang the laundry barefoot, and sat on the sun-hot back steps, pulling burrs out of the soles of my feet.

The house was nestled more or less at the foot of a mountain, Mount Ainslie. The name Canberra is supposed to come from a Ngunnawal word, *kambera*, a meeting place. Much more likely it derives from *nganbira*, the hollow between two breasts, the twin uprising swells of Mount Ainslie and Black Mountain. I like this story better, for the space between the earth's breasts must be more or less directly above her heart. Slow and lean, the trees here rustle in hot north wind, trading secrets in a leaf language of wattle and gum.

This is where I live now, in a state that is betwixt and between; halfway between Melbourne and Sydney, a ready-

made, in the slow big-sky pace of daily life. Outwardly
it is unremarkable—a house in the suburbs, a husband, a
child. But still I catch glimpses of myself as I ride my bike or
water the garden, and marvel that all of this life is mine.

One thing, at least, is evident; I have become a mother.
At three, Owen is beautiful, skinny, and strong, engrossed
in his own private world of animals, insects, rocks, and
stones. Now that Mike is home, Owen can safely ignore
me, unafraid that I, too, will vanish. It is no longer crucial
that I be always in his presence. But where before I was
hands to him, height, essentially a piece of furniture, now
I have been resolved into one coherent image—Mummy.

His eyes, so perfectly blue, follow me across the room;
he flashes me a grin when he catches me looking back
at him. In the morning, he potters around for a while, then
comes to climb into bed with me: "Wake *up*, Mummy!" If
I am reading—and I can read again now—he will insinu-
ate himself into my lap like a cat, wiggling in by degrees
until I can ignore him no longer. "A tickle monster . . . ?"
he asks, hopeful. "A tickle *spider*!" and he giggles and
squirms with delight as my fingertips move across his belly,
my nose pressed into his thicket of fresh, fine hair.

At night I stand in his doorway and watch his little chest
rise and fall, just for a moment, because the fierce rush of
my love for him is almost physically painful. I take in the
thick lashes forming hemispheres on milky, squashy cheeks,
the rosebud pink of his half-open mouth. In the sliver of
light coming from the doorframe, the pale hairs on his legs
are fine as silk, brushing like grass across a plain of scrapes

and bruises. His feet, half off the bed, are Mike's, broad and flat, pink-white toenails like mother-of-pearl. I close the door gently, so as not to wake him up. He is safe, snug, held fast in dreams until the morning comes and the day unfolds again.

The kookaburras raise their voices first, warbling as the first rays of yellow dawn touch the ground. Dozing, I think I can hear bellbirds and wrens, small secret noises that subside in the full scorch of day, when the harsh caw of magpies and galahs cuts across a steady background of cicadas, and tiny lizards streak out from under our terracotta pots. Inside, the sleeping house begins to wake, birdsong merging with the rustle of sheets as Mike turns over in bed, the thump as he plumps up his pillow, Owen's morning chat to the soft toys in his bed.

I dig in the garden, plant basil and parsley. We move the concrete pavers surrounding a heap of dried grass and find rich soil underneath, ready to be turned over into compost. Owen is fascinated by the worm farm, often running out to see it. He holds Bunny up so that Bunny can see. "Hello, worms," they say, and look closely at the wriggling dirt.

I do find the bird book eventually, nestled in with a stack of old poems. What I had thought to be lorikeets among the rosellas are actually their offspring, *Platycercus elegans*. They are "golden-olive with patchy crimson forehead, throat, under-tail coverts; blue cheek-patch, shoulder, blue-white tail edges."[1] Over the summer they will lose their golden-olive plumes and reveal themselves crimson and blue. They take to the wing, startled, as Owen runs out to see them. For a moment he stares at the empty sky. Then he turns toward the next thing, calm and unfazed, small feet padding across the cool, soft earth.

RED LIPS

1. Eliot, T. S. "The Love Song of J. Alfred Prufrock," *Collected Poems 1909–1962*. London: Faber and Faber, 2002.
2. Kristeva, Julia. *The Powers of Horror: An Essay on Abjection*, translated by Leon S. Rudiez. New York: Columbia University Press, 1982.

SWANLIGHTS, *TURNING*

1. An ongoing tally of Australian women killed by male violence is available to the public on Twitter through the Counting Dead Women project, at @DeadWomenAus.
2. Bettelheim, Bruno. *The Uses of Enchantment: The Meaning and Importance of Fairy Tales*. New York: Penguin, 1991.
3. As summarized in Merchant, Carolyn. *The Death of Nature: Women, Ecology, and the Scientific Revolution*. New York: HarperCollins, 1990.
4. Ibid.

5. Antony and the Johnsons. "Her Eyes Are Underneath the Ground." *The Crying Light*, 2009.

6. Antony and the Johnsons. "River of Sorrow." *Antony and the Johnsons*, 2000.

7. Antony and the Johnsons. "Future Feminism." *Cut the World*, 2012.

8. Eliade, Mircea. *Myths, Rites, Symbols: A Mircea Eliade Reader*, edited by Wendell C. Beane and William G. Doty. New York: Harper & Row, 1976.

9. Atlas, Charles and Blair Young. *Turning*, 2012.

10. Cixous, Hélène, and Catherine Clément. *The Newly Born Woman*, translation by Betsy Wing; introduction by Sandra M. Gilbert. Minneapolis: University of Minnesota Press, 1986.

11. Herman, Judith. *Trauma and Recovery: From Domestic Abuse to Political Terror*. New York: Basic Books, 1992.

12. Antony and the Johnsons. "Fistful of Love." *I Am a Bird Now*, 2005.

13. Antony and the Johnsons. "Cripple and the Starfish." *Antony and the Johnsons*, 2000.

14. Antony and the Johnsons. "My Lady Story." *I Am a Bird Now*, 2005.

15. The word *country*, or the phrase "on country," has a particular meaning for Indigenous Australians, set out by the caretakers for Mungo here:

> When Aboriginal people use the English word "Country" it is meant in a special way. For Aboriginal people culture, nature and land are all linked. Aboriginal communities have a cultural connection to the land, which is based on each community's distinct culture, traditions and laws.
>
> Country takes in everything within the landscape— landforms, waters, air, trees, rocks, plants, animals,

foods, medicines, minerals, stories and special places. Community connections include cultural practices, knowledge, songs, stories and art, as well as all people: past, present and future. People have custodial responsibilities to care for their Country, to ensure that it continues in proper order and provides physical sustenance and spiritual nourishment. These custodial relationships may determine who can speak for particular Country.

These concepts are central to Aboriginal spirituality and continue to contribute to Aboriginal identity. Aboriginal communities associate natural resources with the use and benefit of traditional foods and medicines, caring for the land, passing on cultural knowledge and strengthening social bonds.

In the past century, the Australian government has sought to exploit natural resources such as coal and uranium, often for export, without consultation with the Indigenous populations, whose custodial responsibilities this violates. Country is not often recognized by a government that is founded on the idea of terra nullius, and permission for multinational corporations to build mines within Australia continues to be granted, despite Indigenous protest.

16. Antony and the Johnsons, featuring Boy George. "You Are My Sister." *I Am a Bird Now*, 2005.

CENTER STAGE, FIVE DANCES, AND OTHER DANCE ON-SCREEN

1. Quoted in Cvejic, Bojana. *Choreographing Problems: Expressive Concepts in European Contemporary Dance and Performance*. New York: Palgrave Macmillan, 2015.

ALTERED NIGHT

1. Hustvedt, Siri. "Embodied Visions." *Living, Thinking, Looking*. Strongsville, OH: Scepter, 2012.

2. Washington University School of Medicine. "Depression May Shrink Key Brain Structure." *ScienceDaily*, June 16, 1999.

3. Afnan Hamed-Agbariah, Rosenfeld Y. "The Added Value of Art Therapy for Mothers with Postpartum Depression in Arabic Society in Israel." *Harefuah*, September 2015; 154(9):568–72, 608.

4. Barthes, Roland. "Novels and Children." *Mythologies*. Paris: Editions de Seuil, 1957.

5. Fried, Michael. *Art and Objecthood: Essays and Reviews*. Chicago: University of Chicago Press, 1998.

6. Hustvedt, Siri. "Embodied Visions." *Living, Thinking, Looking*. Strongsville, OH: Scepter, 2012.

WEAVING

1. Banks, Lynne Reid. *The Backward Shadow*. Harmondsworth, UK: Penguin Books, 1970.

2. Kruger, Kathryn Sullivan. *Weaving the Word: Metaphorics of Weaving and Female Textual Production*. Plainsboro, NJ: Susquehanna University Press, 2002.

3. Godden, Rumer. *A Time to Dance, No Time to Weep*. London: Macmillan London, 1987.

WALKING

1. Kellerman NP. "Epigenetic Transmission of Holocaust Trauma: Can Nightmares be Inherited?" *Israeli Journal of Psychiatry and Related Sciences* 2013, 50(1):33–9.

2. Foley, Gary. "Australia and the Holocaust: a Koori Perspective." *The Power of Whiteness and Other Essays. Aboriginal Studies Occasional Paper (1)*. Melbourne: Centre for Indigenous Education, University of Melbourne, 1999.

3. *RN Books and Arts*. "New Play explores Aboriginal and Jewish Experience." Segment presented by Michael Cathcart, May 11, 2016.

4. Biss, Eula. "White Debt: Reckoning What Is Owed—and

Can Never be Repaid—for Racial Privilege." *The New York Times Magazine*, December 2, 2015.

5. According to OxfordDictionaries.com, a songline is "a route through the landscape which is believed to have been travelled during the Dreamtime and which features a series of landmarks thought to relate to events that happened during this time."

Intricate phrasing and changes in rhythm and tone in these sung routes, as well as their words, allow the singer to navigate the terrain; their melodic contours map the landscape, even across language groups. In this way a singer can cross terrain he has never before seen.

Songlines also carry sacred knowledge, which custodians hold and protect. Many songlines are in danger of disappearing, as elders approach the end of their lives with nobody to entrust their knowledge to. This is one of the many traumas of settler-colonialism.

6. Jack, Dana Crowley, and Ali, Alishia (eds). *Silencing the Self Across Cultures: Depression and Gender in the Social World*. London: Oxford University Press, 2010.

7. The Australian edition of this book went to print around the time of Trump's inauguration; I am looking at these words, six months later, in order to make revisions for an American readership, and reading at the same time in the news about synagogue services in Texas that have gone underground for fear of neo-Nazi attack. In fact we do not say "neo-Nazi" anymore; the armies of Trump-styled white men who have assembled in the streets of Charlottesville are named as Nazis, nothing less. It is Rosh Hashanah today, and I am trying to navigate a world in which White Supremacists chant "Jews will not replace us!" as they attempt to beat the shit out of black bodies in full daylight, aware that there will be no consequences.

While the anti-Semitic rhetoric and hatred has come out of hiding, and while it is almost a relief to put an end to the gaslighting, the feeling of paranoia, it is still overwhelmingly black bodies that are most directly affected by physical and structural violence, even when it is our name that is being invoked. The situation for non-Ashkenazi Jews, black Jews, and the Mizrahi and people of color must be almost unbearable. I don't want to see what the next month brings, let alone the New Year—but I have baked an apple cake anyway, and let my son lick the spoon—and hope that all of us can have a moment of peace, of rest, before the onslaught begins again. *L'shanah tova* to anyone reading this endnote, and may the work of our next year be an attempt to disentangle ourselves from a hierarchy that offers us only conditional acceptance, and to throw ourselves into a social justice in which black lives matter.

8. I learned of these cycles as an adult, and immediately wondered why I hadn't known about them as a child. Owen will have better knowledge, though: the Bureau of Meteorology has been incorporating Indigenous Weather Knowledge into its forecasts since 2002, and now gives information on a dozen weather systems around the country.

9. Steinlauf, Gil. "Jews in America Struggled for Decades to Become White. Now We Must Give Up Whiteness to Fight Racism." *Washington Post*, September 22, 2015.

RINGS

1. Nin, Anaïs. *In Favor of the Sensitive Man and Other Essays.* New York: Mariner Books, 1976.

AINSLIE

1. Knight, Frank, and Pizzey, Graham. "Crimson Rosella." *The Field Guide to the Birds of Australia.* Sydney: Angus & Robertson, 1997.

ACKNOWLEDGMENTS

When I began writing these essays, I felt as though I was picking through the charred ruins of a house fire, looking for valuables; but the writing itself soon became what was most precious about the exercise. I feel very, very grateful to have been given the opportunity to make this work.

Many thanks to the friends and family who have lent their support over the past few years. Some appear in these pages, some do not; but every coffee, every text and phone call, and every act of kindness and silliness and love has been deeply appreciated. A special thanks to those who read early drafts or hashed out ideas over dinner, particularly Ming-Zhu Hii and Geoff Lemon for their thoughtful engagement and nice words.

The writing of this book was partly funded by Creative

Victoria; they awarded the grant mentioned on page 229, and I am very appreciative of their faith in me. The book's completion would not have been possible without the wonderful, incisive, and gentle Marika Webb-Pullman, and the extended family at Scribe. I also wish to thank Grace Heifetz and Allison Colpoys, who round out a trio of amazing women whose cheerleading for the project bolstered me greatly.

Though this book is dedicated to my mother, there are three other people without whom it would not have been possible: the remarkable Kristy-Anne Adnams, who helped make sense of so much; and Mike and Owen, my beautiful boys. Every day you bring me so much joy. I can't wait to see what the next years hold.